PHYSIOLOGY AND PHARMACOLOGY OF CARDIO-RESPIRATORY CONTROL

PHYSIOLOGY AND PHARMACOLOGY OF CARDIO-RESPIRATORY CONTROL

Edited by

Albert Dahan
Leiden University Medical Center, Leiden, The Netherlands

Luc Teppema
Leiden University Medical Center, Leiden, The Netherlands

and

Johannes H.G.M. van Beek
Free University, Amsterdam, The Netherlands

KLUWER ACADEMIC PUBLISHERS
DORDRECHT / BOSTON / LONDON

A C.I.P. Catalogue record for this book is available from the Library of Congress.

ISBN 0-7923-5135-5

Published by Kluwer Academic Publishers,
P.O. Box 17, 3300 AA Dordrecht, The Netherlands.

Sold and distributed in North, Central and South America
by Kluwer Academic Publishers,
101 Philip Drive, Norwell, MA 02061, U.S.A.

In all other countries, sold and distributed
by Kluwer Academic Publishers,
P.O. Box 322, 3300 AH Dordrecht, The Netherlands.

Printed on acid-free paper

Cover:
Fractal branching structure mimicking bronchial or blood vessel tree,
generated with an L-system program on the computer.

Printed in the Netherlands

Contents

List of contributors

J. G. van den Aardweg
    Department of Pulmonology
    Leiden University Medical Center
    2300 RC Leiden, The Netherlands

J. H. G. M. van Beek
    Laboratory for Physiology
    Institute for Cardiovascular Research
    Vrije Universiteit, Amsterdam

F. Boer
    Department of Anesthesiology
    Leiden University Medical Center
    2300 RC Leiden, The Netherlands

J. M. Bogaard
    Department of Pulmonary Diseases
    Erasmus University Rotterdam
    3015 GD Rotterdam, The Netherlands

J. G. Bovill
    Department of Anesthesiology
    Leiden University Medical Center
    2300 RC Leiden, The Netherlands

A. Dahan
    Departments of Anesthesiology and Physiology
    Leiden University Medical Center
    2300 RC Leiden, The Netherlands

G. B. Drummond
    Department of Anaesthetics
    Royal Infirmary
    Edinburgh EH3 9YW, Scotland

H. Folgering
    Department of Pulmonology Dekkerswald
    University of Nijmegen, The Netherlands

D. Gozal
    Constance S. Kaufman Pediatric Research Laboratory
    Departments of Pediatrics and Physiology
    Tulane University School of Medicine
    New Orleans, Louisiana 70112, USA

C. P. M. van der Grinten
    Department of Pulmonology
    Academic Hospital Maastricht
    6206 AZ Maastricht, The Netherlands

Y. Heijdra
    Department of Pulmonology Dekkerswald
    University of Nijmegen, The Netherlands

C. van Herwaarden
    Department of Pulmonology Dekkerswald
    University of Nijmegen, The Netherlands

Y. Honda
    Department of Physiology
    School of Medicine
    Chiba University
    Chiba, 260 Japan

J. R.C. Jansen
    Pathophysiology Laboratory
    Department of Pulmonary Diseases
    Erasmus University Rotterdam
    3015 GD Rotterdam, The Netherlands

J. M. Karemaker
    Department of Physiology
    Academic Medical Center
    Amsterdam, The Netherlands

B. Kest
    Department of Psychology
    The Collge of Staten Island
    City University of New York
    Staten Island, New York 10314, USA

H. Kimura
Department of Chest Medicine
School of Medicine
Chiba University
Chiba, 260 Japan

T. Kobayashi
Department of Physiology
School of Medicine, Chiba University
Chiba, 260 Japan

J. A. Kuipers
Department of Anesthesiology
Leiden University Medical Center
2300 RC Leiden, The Netherlands

T. Kuriyama
Department of Chest Medicine
School of Medicine, Chiba University
Chiba, 260 Japan

S. C. M. Luijendijk
Department of Pulmonology
Academic Hospital Maastricht
6206 AZ Maastricht, The Netherlands

S. Masuyama
Department of Chest Medicine
School of Medicine, Chiba University
Chiba, 260 Japan

A. Masuda
Department of Physiology
School of Medicine, Chiba University
Chiba, 260 Japan

A. Mizoo
Department of Chest Medicine
School of Medicine, Chiba University
Chiba, 260 Japan

J. S. Mogil
Department of Psychology
Univ of Illinois at Urbana-Champaign
Champaign, Illinois 61820, USA

K. Nagano
    Department of Chest Medicine
    School of Medicine, Dokkyo University Hospital
    Koshigaya, 343 Japan

M. Niijima
    Department of Chest Medicine
    School of Medicine, Chiba University
    Chiba, 260 Japan

E. Olofsen
    Department of Anesthesiology
    Leiden University Medical Center
    2300 RC Leiden, The Netherlands

B. Oeseburg
    Department of Physiology
    Faculty of Medical Sciences
    University of Nijmegen
    6500 HB Nijmegen, The Netherlands

C. N. Olievier
    Department of Physiology
    Leiden University Medical Center
    2300 RC Leiden, The Netherlands

P. A. Robbins
    The University Laboratory of Physiology
    Parks Road
    Oxford OX1 3PT, UK

E. Y. Sarton
    Department of Anesthesiology
    Leiden University Medical Center
    2300 RC Leiden, The Netherlands

J. W. Severinghaus
    Department of Anesthesiology
    University of California San Fransisco
    San Fransisco, California 94143, USA

R. P. van Steenwijk
    Department of Pulmonology
    Academic Medical Center
    Amsterdam

M. Tanaka
Department of Physiology
School of Medicine, Chiba University
Chiba, 260 Japan

K Tatsumi
Department of Chest Medicine
School of Medicine, Chiba University
Chiba, 260 Japan

L. J. Teppema
Department of Anesthesiology
Leiden University Medical Center
2300 RC Leiden, The Netherlands

T. Uruma
Department of Chest Medicine
School of Medicine, Chiba University
Chiba, 260 Japan

J. G. Veening
Department of Anantomy and Embryology
University of Nijmegen
Nijmegen, The Netherlands

A. Versprille
Pathophysiology Laboratory
Department of Pulmonary Diseases
Erasmus University Rotterdam
3015 GD Rotterdam

P. Vos
Department of Pulmonology Dekkerswald
University of Nijmegen
The Netherlands

M. Wagenaar
Department of Pulmonology Dekkerswald
University of Nijmegen
The Netherlands

D. S. Ward
Departments of Anesthesiology and Electrical Engineering
University of Rochester
Rochester, New York 14642, USA

P. M. Warren
    Respiratory Medicine Unit
    The University of Edinburgh
    Edinburgh EH3 9YW, Scotland

P. K. Wraith
    Department of Medical Physics
    Royal Infirmary of Ediburgh Trust
    Edinburgh EH3 9YW, Scotland

Preface

On 15 November 1997, the first international symposium "Neural and Chemical Control of Breathing: Pharmacological and Clinical Aspects" was held at Leiden University Medical Center on the occasion of the retirement of one of the members of the Control of Breathing Research Group of the Departments of Physiology and Anesthesiology, Dr. Aad Berkenbosch. Among others, Dr. Berkenbosch, played an important role in this research group, which made a large and significant contribution to scientific research on the regulation of breathing. This book presents the proceedings of that meeting together with papers of several authors who have strong bonds with the Leiden Departments of Physiology and Anesthesiology. All studies represent state of the art work on the subject of respiratory control and cardiovascular medicine, with emphasis on the physiological, pharmacological and anesthesiological aspects of both fields.

The book is divided in several sections:

Oxygen Physiology. Prof. John Severinghaus presents among other things his ideas on oxygen sensing and high altitude related diseases. Prof. Honda gives results from studies in a unique set of subjects without carotid bodies. The findings of Honda's group support the idea that an intact hypoxic drive from the carotid bodies is necessary for the generation of central hypoxic depression. Dr. Hans van Beek discusses the effects of hypoxia and hypercapnia on cardiac contractility in animal models. Prof. Oeseburg demonstrates the feasibility of Near Infra Red Oximetry for monitoring tissue oxygenation in patients.

Central Chemoreception. Two active members of the Control of Breathing Research Group from Leiden, Dr. Luc Teppema and Kees Olievier, present recent work on the identification of structures in the brainstem responding to hypercapnia (central chemoreceptors ?) with the use of the technique of *c-fos* immunochemistry and on the importance of brain blood flow induced reduction of brain PCO_2 in the development of ventilatory decline due to long-term hypoxia in an anesthetized cat model.

Breathing Disorders in Wakefulness and Sleep. Several respiratory diseases are discussed in relation to central and peripheral control: asthma, COPD, sleep apnea syndrome and the congenital hypoventilation syndrome.

Artificial Ventilation. The influence of alternating ventilation of the two lungs on hemodynamics in a pig model is discussed by researchers from the Erasmus University.

Opioids and Anesthetics. Prof. Jim Bovill discusses the influence of endogenous and exogenously administered opioids on the heart and the hemodynamics of cerebral and peripheral vessels; Prof. Denham Ward reviews the influence of inhalational anesthetics on ventilatory control in relation to their mechanisms of action; Dr. Gordon Drummond

1

2

presents recent work on the influence of opioids on abdominal muscle action. Furthermore, the differential effects of opioids on analgesia and respiration in men and women are reviewed by authors from Staten Island College, University of Illinois and Leiden University Medical Center. This is an interesting and fashionable field of research which, until recently, obtained only little attention from physiologists and anesthesiologists. Dr. Albert Dahan pays tribute to the late Prof. Richard Knill from London, Ontario. Prof. Knill was one of the first to study the influence of anesthetics on ventilatory control in volunteers and patients. His pioneering and unique work has been the basis of many of the studies performed by the Leiden Control of Breathing Research Group in animals and human volunteers.

Modeling Studies. This section represents the large interest from basic scientists (pharmacologists and physiologists) and clinicians (anesthesiologists) in modeling pharmacological and physiological responses. In this section, we find a pharmacokinetic model which is used to improve outcome of pharmacological end-points, an empirical model on the influence of inhalational anesthetics on breathing, which may be used to predict respiration during and immediately after anesthesia, models of the ventilatory response to hypoxia, a mathematical exercise on the interaction between carbon dioxide and hypoxia on ventilation and, finally, a study that shows the inadequacy of rebreathing technique in the assessment of the ventilatory response to carbon dioxide.

This book is a unique collection of state of the art studies and reviews which are of interest to basic scientists and clinicians with interest in ventilatory control, cardio-respiratory physiology, breathing disorders, anesthesia and analgesia and modeling. It shows that integrative cardio-respiratory physiology, together with molecular and cellular biochemical sciences will continue to aid clinicians at the bedside and in the operating room.

Finally, we would like to acknowledge Datex-Engstrom BV. Their generous financial support made the publication of this book possible.

Albert Dahan
Luc Teppema
Leiden, April 1998

Hans van Beek
Amsterdam, April 1998

Enigmas and insights in the oxybiology of high altitude

John W. Severinghaus

Introduction

Aad Berkenbosch and I are near the end of long careers in respiratory physiology, in which we both have puzzled over some of the unknowns and mysteries of oxy-biology. It seems of use as well as interest to examine these areas in which the next generation may find fertile ground for their research and application of so many new skills and methods, even if, to do so, we need to look so far back in our own experiences as to suggest total obsolescence in what we say.

The study of oxygen is at the base of all physiology, and its mysteries are among the most important for our understanding of our bodies. My perspective of oxygen reactions is colored by a background in physics and physical chemistry, particularly in the understanding of polarographic oxygen electrodes, and the 35 year effort in my laboratory to understand the impact of high altitude on climbers and sojourners. I thus may draw different schemes than are common among biochemists. For many years, some of the mechanisms involving oxygen in physiology have intruiged me Let us call them enigmas. Here I take the prerogative of this forum to present speculative insights into problems associated with high altitude work, a few of which may even be true!

I. Carotid body

Enigmas: How can the carotid body sense arterial Po_2, not oxygen content of blood or blood saturation considering its very high metabolic rate? How can the response to hypoxia be generated as a nearly linear function of hemoglobin desaturation? What is the normal Po_2 at the sensing site in the neurone? How does chronic hypoxia have a three phase effect: 1) To cause at least a doubling of the sensitivity of the peripheral chemoreceptors to hypoxia within a week or two; 2) To lead to hypertrophy of the carotid bodies; and 3) To slowly result in decay or "blunting" of the ventilatory response to hypoxia?

Insights: I draw on my 40 years of work with polarographic oxygen electrodes for an insight into the first enigma, the insensitivity of the carotid body response to blood O_2 content. Electrodes consume all the oxygen reaching the metalic surface. A semipermeable membrane (e.g. polypropylene) separates metal from sample, and confines most of the O_2 gradient within itself. However, all electrodes have a stirring effect, i.e. the current increases if the sample is flowing.[1] This effect defeated attempts to calibrate early electrodes covered with cellophane, became a manageable 10-15% stirring effect with Leland Clark's first electrode in which a 2 mm diameter platinum cathode was covered with polyethylene, and was finally made almost negligible by reducing cathode diameter to 10 microns, and using less permeable polypropylene. In the case of the carotid body, blood flows through sinusoids at high velocity, rather than through capillaries.[2] It is therefore reasonable to postulate that the surface stirring of this high flow keeps the PO_2 at the endothelial surface equal to arterial PO_2, independent of the presence of hemoglobin in the blood, and despite the very high metabolic rate of the sensory cells. The lack of an effect of blood O_2 content has usually been attributed to separation of plasma from red cells by streaming, but no such mechanism is needed at high flow rate. Further confirmation is that carotid bodies are stimulated by hypotension and reduced flow.[2] The stimulus due to locally injected vasodilators such as papaverine[3] suggest that shunts open which reduce flow velocity past the critical sensory endothelial surfaces. The very high metabolic rate of the mammalian carotid body generates a diffusion gradient within the tissue.[4] A long-standing target of much research has been to determine the PO_2 in the sensory mechanism. Microelectrode studies in the carotid body have reported both very low and almost arterial values. This concept is still unresolved, and perhaps cannot be expected to help if the O_2 gradients are steep immediately around the sites of high consumption.

There may be a useful insight reached by taking a different approach which can suggest an answer to both the above enigmas, the apparent linearity with blood O_2 saturation, and the unknown internal PO_2. The logic is as follows: the response plot has long been called hyperbolic, with a low PO_2 asymptote of about 30 mmHg. Like other highly active tissues (e.g. brain) O_2 consumption may be assumed to be independent of PO_2 over a wide range, down to some critical threshold PO_2, below which consumption falls as a linear function proportional to PO_2. For many tissues this threshold is about 30 mmHg. At this critical threshold the PO_2 at the cytochrome surface may be assumed to have reached zero, all the delivered O_2 being consumed on arrival. Like an O_2 electrode, which always operates with zero PO_2 at the metal surface, the consumption in this lower range becomes proportional to the PO_2 at the membrane's external surface, or the endothelial surface. This logic suggests that the normal carotid body should have a gradient due to its own metabolic rate of about 30 mmHg between blood and cytochrome. With falling PO_2, the gradient remains about 30 mmHg until P_aO_2 reaches 30, and cytochrome reaches zero. In the actual heterogeneous situation, some of the aa_3 metal reaches zero PO_2 early, so the transition would not be perfectly abrupt.

If O_2 consumption is constant over this wide range down to 30 mmHg, what produces the signal? The answer is similar to that applying to skeletal muscle, as described below:[5] As PO_2 falls from above normal but far above the critical PO_2 (e.g. 30 mmHg), the redox state of the mitochondria gradually is reduced because the scarcer O_2 molecules at the surface result in accumulation of electrons waiting to reduce an O_2 molecule. When P_aO_2 is less than 30, no further reduction occurs because at 30 mmHg, the cytochrome is fully reduced, the PO_2 at the sensory site (probably a K^+ channel) has reached zero, hence no further increase in neural output would be expected. This model nicely accounts then for both enigmas, the hyperbolic response and the independence of blood O_2 carrying capacity.

How then does the response appear linear with hemoglobin desaturation? The upper portion of the O_2 dissociation curve can be approximated by a hyperbola (Figure 1). The scarce data on this relationship in man suggests that below 70%, the response is more than a linear relationship to desaturation would predict, but in accord with the concept that the carotid body stimulus is a hyperbolic function of P_{O_2}.[6]

Carotid body type I "neurosecretory" cells (the presumed chemoreceptors) have O_2 sensitive K^+ channels believed to be involved in O_2 detection.[7,8] Hypoxia inhibits outward K^+ currents in these cells, reducing their membrane potential toward the firing threshold. O_2 sensing by these channels involves an iron protein (not heme) in CNS neurones.[8,9] This iron protein is present even in cell free patches of membrane, and must be attached to or close by the K^+ channel. Similar hypoxia sensitive K^+ channels are found in pulmonary arterioles and in carotid body glomus cells, and both appear dependent upon the redox state of the cell.[9] However, the high metabolic rate in carotid body reduces P_{O_2} at the sensory channel while no such reduction is known to occur in pulmonary arterioles.

II. Pulmonary arteries

Enigmas: What mechanism permits the pulmonary arterioles to respond to falling P_{O_2} at levels of oxygen tension in the normal sea level range, making it more sensitive than the carotid body, despite absence of any cells with high metabolic rate? What mechanism can explain the strong evidence that HAPE is coupled to pulmonary arterial hypertension, not capillary hypertension? How can pulmonary vasodilators (eg nifedipine) ameliorate hypoxically induced pulmonary edema if the leakage is downstream from the pulmonary arterioles? Can periarterial cuffs of edema and red cells be explained by lymphatic carriage from alveolar capillary extracellular space. If so, how can this occur in hypoxic but not left heart failure types of pulmonary edema?

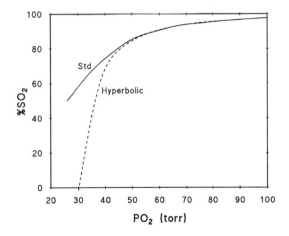

Figure 1. The peripheral chemoreceptor response to hypoxia appears to be a linear function of arterial oxygen desaturation down to 70% largely because its hyperbolic response can mimic the oxygen dissociation curve of normal humans down to that level. At lower saturation, carotid body output rises hyperbolically, which provokes a greater ventilatory response than would be expected if it were a function of desaturation.

Insights: The response of smooth muscles in pulmonary arteries is an S shaped curve like a dissociation curve of blood, but with a half constriction P_{50} of about 60 mmHg, compared with blood P_{50} of 27 mmHg.[10] Sensitivity to these relatively high levels of oxygen without a site of high metabolic rate has been an enigma, but now evidence for neuro-epithelial bodies scattered throughout the airway, with histologic characteristics of carotid body[11] and potassium channel responses to hypoxia similar to those of carotid body glomus cells, suggests a mechanism for HPV.[12] The inherent sensitivity must, however, differ from those of carotid body, and it is not at all clear whether some unusual cytochrome in pulmonary arterioles (e.g. a P_{450} with a half saturation PO_2 of 60 mmHg) generates their response at such high PO_2.

High altitude pulmonary edema (HAPE) is caused by pulmonary arterial (not capillary) hypertension, is readily prevented or treated by pulmonary vasodilation with nifedipine or NO.[13] HAPE is first detectable as perihilar fuzziness around major vessels. Sputum protein concentration is that of plasma indicating large cracks rather than Starling type filtration (as in cardiac failure). The major pulmonary arteries can rupture in horses during racing at high altitude (Hultgren, personal comm.). Acute hypoxia with catecholamine release may cause a similar syndrome at sea level, e.g. heroin overdose, respiratory disconnect in awake paralyzed subjects, and post anesthetic airway obstruction, especially in muscular young men. In addition, there may be a link to respiratory infections, and to VEGF of angiogenesis (see brain below) since lung tissue VEGF concentration is very high in experimental hypoxia in rats. This and other evidence suggested to me that the damage is thus most probably due to over-distension damage to the walls of the highly distensible, elastic, large pulmonary arteries which serve as reservoirs for the stroke volume, permitting leakage into the periarterial cuffs which are seen both on X-ray and histologically (in animal models).[14,15] This hypothesis, which has been considered by others for some 25 years, remains controversial and largely ignored in favor of capillary stress failure,[16] for which evidence is minimal.

III. Skeletal muscles

Enigmas: Why do muscles generate lactate at high work rate even when O_2 consumption and aerobic ATP production continue to match work rate? How does hypoxia have such profound biochemical effects without a decrease in O_2 consumption? How can the cytochrome PO_2 be zero at VO_2max? And how can muscle myoglobin oxygen saturation fall to about 50% with mild exercise, and not fall farther with maximum work rate?

Insights: The physiologic cause that limits exercise has not been identified. However, by analogy with O_2 electrodes, it can be shown that all studies of capillary PO_2 and O_2 consumption are consistent with the hypothesis that PO_2 at the cytochromes falls to zero at VO_2max, from which a generalization is appropriate: Exercise is limited by O_2 delivery, ceasing at the point at which all the O_2 which can be extracted from passing blood is being consumed. At the cytochrome surface, there are sufficient electrons available such than no O_2 molecules remain unreduced, i.e. $PO_2 = 0$.[5]

As work increases, or if hypoxia occurs, in order for O_2 consumption to equal the flux of electrons (i.e. reducing equivalents, or metabolites), as the number of O_2 molecules at or near the cytochrome surface falls, the number of electrons must rise (this is the mass law). The accumulation of electrons in hypoxia is seen as a redox reduction, with which the concentrations of each of the metabolic intermediates in the citric acid cycle increases. The rise in pyruvate results in a rise in tissue lactate, and diffusion of this lactate out to blood as long as blood concentration of La is lower than tissue concentration. This outward diffusion is commonly called anaerobic metabolism, despite the direct proportionality of O_2 consumption to work rate (showing that work is actually still essentially fully aerobic. The ATP generated by increasing lactate generation is almost a negligible fraction of total energy production. The more important function of the lactic acid is to acidify blood and raise PO_2.[17]

Muscle venous PO_2 in exercise falls to about 15 mm Hg at about 60% of VO_2max, but falls no further at higher work rate due to lactic acidification of blood shifting the O_2 dissociation curve rightward, i.e. raising blood PO_2 at given saturation.[17] Muscle venous blood saturation can fall below 10%. VO_2max is directly proportional to venous PO_2 in subjects breathing low vs normal O_2 during exercise.[18]

IV. Brain effects of hypoxia (AMS, HACE)

Enigmas: What causes brain and retinal blood vessels to leak at high altitude? What permits tolerance to more severe hypoxia after a few days of acclimatization and/or recovery? Does hypoxia injure neurones directly or only by interference with blood supply through either local hemorrhage and compression, or through systemic hypotension? Is brain injury in mountaineers more in those who have higher blood O_2 and lower blood PCO_2 levels?

Insights: The several formerly proposed mechanisms underlying HACE have not stood the tests of time or experiment. HACE is not due to either high cerebral blood flow or lack of ATP. Some mechanism must account for the petechial hemorrhages seen in the retina. A new candidate is the process of angiogenesis.[19] As tissues grow or become hypoxia, the cells attract macrophages which express an mRNA followed within 3-12 hours by VEGF (vascular endothelial growth factor), also known as VPF, (vascular permeability factor), a protein cytokine which dissolves basement membranes of capillaries, permitting the endothelial junctions to break, plasma and red cells to leak out, and later, with help of other angiogenesis factors, facilitating growth of capillary tubules into hypoxic (growing or infarcted) tissue. This first stage of angiogenesis is blocked by dexamethazone, which is used both to slow cancer tissue growth, and to prevent or treat acute mountain sickness and high altitude cerebral edema. This supports the concept that HACE is due to this VEGF attack during the first step of angiogenesis.

I have suggested that two other contributory mechanisms may be involved in HACE.[19] 1) Hypoxia immediately increases cell water osmotically as anaerobic glucose breakdown increases concentration of each substrate both within and outside of mitochondria. 2) Acute hypoxic lactic acid generation may titrate tissue HCO_3^- stores, raising tissue PCO_2. At altitude, total tissue gas pressure is not lower than ambient (whereas at sea level tissue is about 50 mm Hg below ambient). If gas microbubbles are present or occur, at altitude their growth would be facilitated by the higher than ambient total pressure. Among climbers and high altitude physicians there is a significant impression that either descent or increased pressure using a Gamow bag provides relief more rapidly than breathing oxygen in subjects with HACE, and this, if true, could only be explained by the presence of gas microbubbles in the brain.

Climbers who have strong hypoxic ventilatory responses breathe more deeply at altitude and thus are better oxygenated, but they have been suggested to suffer more permanent (tested at 6 mo) loss of certain subtle brain functions (number memory, finger tapping speed, etc). The hypothetic mechanism is hypocapnic cerebral vasoconstriction, not hypoxemia itself.[20]

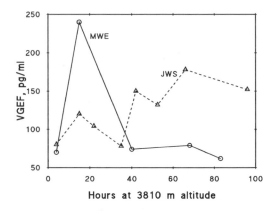

Figure 2. The concentration of Vascular Endothelial Growth Factor, step 1 of angiogenesis, rose in two subjects at high altitude, but fell promptly to normal in the younger subject who did not experience nose bleeding, and continued to rise in the older subject who did experience bleeding. VEGF dissolves capillary basement membranes, permitting petechial bleeding, here, presumably, in the nasal mucosa.

V. Surface tissue sensitivity to hypoxia
Enigmas: What makes the nasal mucosa so sensitive to hypoxia? The observation of common nosebleeding during the first week at altitudes of 3-5 Km ft is unexplained, but commonly assumed to be due to dryness (although bleeding is not common with sojournes in desert areas).

Insights: Like skin, it is probable that surface layers of nasal mucosa obtain their metabolic oxygen from the ambient air rather than from blood. There should be a vulnerable layer of deeper cells which are normally marginally supplied with oxygen, but which at altitude are too deep to get oxygen through the living more superficial layers. This deeper layer, becoming anoxic, may invoke an angiogenesis response in which VEGF causes local mucosal bleeding. To test this, we obtained nasal washings on two subjects during 4 days at 3810 m altitude, and showed that VEGF concentration rose on the first day in both subjects (Figure 2). It rapidly returned to normal in MWE, who experienced no nose bleeding, but remained elevated in me and I did have bleeding. We conclude that nose bleeds are a result of angiogenic VEGF released in deeper layers of nasal mucosa at altitude.

References

1. Severinghaus JW, Bradley AF Jr. Electrodes for blood P_{O_2} and P_{CO_2} determination. *J Appl Physiol* 13: 515-520, 1958

2. McDonald, DM. Peripheral Chemoreceptors. In: *Regulation of Respiration Part I*. Edited by Hornbein TF.. *Vol 17, Lung Biology in Health and Disease*. Edited by Lenfant C. New York, Dekker, pp 105-319, 1981.

3. Nims RG, Severinghaus JW, Comroe JH Jr. Reflex hyperpnea induced by papaverine acting upon the carotid and aortic body. *J Pharm Exp Therap* 109: 58-61, 1953.

4. Acker H, Lübbers DW. Relationshipbetween local flow, tissue P_{O_2} and total flow of the cat carotid body. In: *Chemoreception in the Carotid Body*. Edited by Acker H. New York, Springer-Verlag, pp 271-276, 1977.

5. Severinghaus JW. Exercise O_2 transport model assuming zero cytochrome P_{O_2} at VO_2max. *J Appl Physiol* 77: 671-678, 1994.

6. Sato M, Severinghaus JW, Powell FL, Xu F, Spellman MJ Jr. Augmented hypoxic ventilatory response in man at altitude. *J Appl Physiol* 73: 101-107, 1992.

7. Ganfornina MD, Lopez-Barneo J. Potassium channel types in arterial chemoreceptor cells and their selective modulation by oxygen. *J Gen Physiol* 100 :401-426, 1992.

8. Jiang C, Haddad GG. A direct mechanism for sensing low oxygen levels by central neurons. *Proc Nat Acad Sci* 91: 7198-7201, 1994.

9. Wyatt CN, Wright C, Bee D, Peers C. O_2-sensitive K^+ currents in carotid body chemoreceptor cells from normoxic and chronically hypoxic rats and their roles in hypoxic chemotransduction *Proc Nat Acad Sci* 92: 295-9 1995.

10. Barer GR, Howard P, Shaw JW. Stimulus-response curves for the pulmonary vascular bed to hypoxia and hypercapnia. *J Physiol Lond* 211: 139, 1970.
    Youngson C, Nurse C, Yeger H, Cutz E. Oxygen sensing in airway chemoreceptors. *Nature* 365: 153-155, 1993.

11. Weir EK, Archer SL. The mechanism of acute hypoxic pulmonary vasoconstriction: the tale of two channels. *FASEB Journal* 9: 183-189, 1995.

12. Scherrer U, Vollenweider L, Delabays A. Inhaled nitric oxide for high altitude pulmonary edema. *N Eng J Med* 334: 624-629, 1996.

13. Severinghaus JW. Pulmonary vascular function. *Am Rev Resp Dis* 115:149-158, 1977.

14. Jerome EH, Severinghaus JW. High altitude pulmonary edema. *N Eng J Med* 334: 662-663, 1996.

15. West JB, Tsukimoto K, Mathieu-Costello O, Prediletto R. Stress failure in pulmonary capillaries. *J Appl Physiol* 70: 1731-1742, 1991.

16. Wasserman K. Coupling of external to cellular respiration during exercise: the wisdom of the body revisited. *Am J Physiol* 266: E519-E539, 1994.

17. Wagner PD, Roca J, Hogan MC, Poole DC, Bebout DE, Haab P. Experimental support for the theory of diffusion limitation of maximum oxygen uptake. *Adv Exp Med Biol* 227: 825-833, 1990.

18. Severinghaus JW. Hypothetic roles of osmotic pressure and angiogenesis in high altitude cerebral edema. *J Appl Physiol* 79:375-379, 1995.
19. Hornbein TF, Townes BD, Schoene RB, Sutton JR, Houston CS. The cost to the central nervous system of climbing to extremely high altitude: *N Eng J Med* 321: 1714-1719, 1989.

Possible role of the carotid body responsible for hypoxic ventilatory decline in awake humans

H. Kimura, M. Tanaka, K. Nagano, M. Niijima, S. Masuyama, A. Mizoo,
T. Uruma, K. Tatsumi, T. Kuriyama, A. Masuda, T. Kobayashi and Y. Honda

Introduction

The carotid body (CB) is the most important chemoreceptor for eliciting hyperpnea in response to hypoxic exposure.[1] However, the level of hypoxic hyperventilation is not maintained at a constant level: ventilation (V_I) during sustained mild hypoxia initially increases rapidly, and then gradually declines with time.[2-4] The initial rapid rise is generally considered to be induced by CB excitation, whereas the mechanism for the subsequent gradual decline (hypoxic ventilatory decline, HVD) is a matter of controversy.[5-9] It has also been confirmed in humans as well as in other animal species that the magnitude of the initial ventilatory increment is closely correlated with secondary HVD.[10-13] Fig. 1 illustrates an example of such a finding previously obtained by us.[13] This fact led us to assume that this specific profile of hypoxic hyperpnea is possibly entirely related to the CB activity. Therefore, we intended to study CB-resected patients who underwent a therapeutic surgery for bronchial asthma some 40 yrs ago. We found that these patients revealed no HVD.

Methods

Three patients with bilateral and one patient with unilateral CB resection (termed BR and UR, respectively) were examined. Forced expiratory flow volume in 1 sec ($FEV_{1.0}$) and blood gas were somewhat depressed, but vital capacity and blood pH were well within normal range. None of the four patients suffered an asthmatic attack during the course of the study and tolerated the examination without complaint. When studied, none of the patients was administering the drugs possibly affecting HVD, such as theophylline. Their operation was carried out as early as during the late 40's to middle 50's. Accordingly, despite of our best effort during last 10 yrs, we were not able to obtain more patients for the present study. The details of the experimental procedure was already described (see ref. 14). Briefly, the subjects breathed through a mouthpiece and a respiratory valve to which a rebreathing circuit was connected. The degree of hypoxemia measured by a pulse oximeter was maintained around 80% in arterial oxygen saturation (SPO_2). It lasted for 16 to 20 min. Tidal volume and airway PO_2 and PCO_2 were continuously measured.

Sleep studies were additionally performed in BR patients N.K. and M.I. SPO_2, respiratory movement measured by an inductance plethysmography (Respitrace®, Ambulatory Monitoring), Electroencephalogram (EEG), Electroocculogram (EOG), Electromyogram (EMG) of the genioglossal muscle recorded by a surface electrode, and Electrocardiogram (ECG) were continuously monitored. In the latter patient, the effect of

11

hypoxia by introducing N_2 gas by a nasal catheter was further examined.

Results

Fig. 2 shows the time course of V_I of all three BR- and one UR-patients expressed in % value relative to the control magnitude. For comparison, the results obtained from 16 normal subjects from our previous study are also added.[13] The Specific profile of hypoxic ventilatory responses, i.e. initial rapid rise followed by gradual decay (termed Biph.HVD), is clearly seen in the control subjects and the UR patient still shows the same profile although only to a lesser degree. It was further noted that the patient exhibited even less than control pre-hypoxic ventilation in the late period, which is often seen in neonates and other animals with weak ventilatory response to hypoxia.[10] In contrast, all three BR patients exhibited neither initial hyperventilation nor its secondary decline. Rather, V_I tended to slightly increase towards the end of hypoxia.

Both BR patients, N.K. and M.I. exhibited no marked respiratory disturbance with room air breathing during sleep. However, when the amount of N_2 gas, given by nasal catheter, increased up to 1.5 l/min during slow wave sleep, severe arterial desaturation developed with apneic episodes as shown in Fig. 3. No such disturbance was detected during light non-REM and REM sleep with the same amount of N_2 administration.

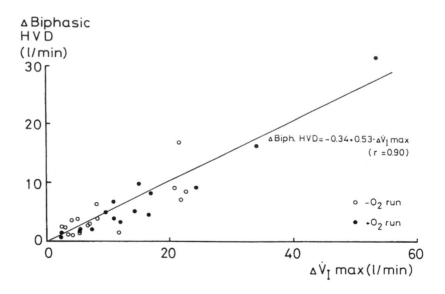

Figure 1. Relationship between initial ventilatory augmentation (ΔV_I max) and the amount of subsequent ventilatory decline (ΔBiphasic HVD) during sustained, isocapnic and mild hypoxia in 16 normal healthy subjects. Good linear correlation was found (r=0.9). ○ response following room air breathing. ● response after prior O_2 breathing. This figure is constructed from the data of ref. 13.

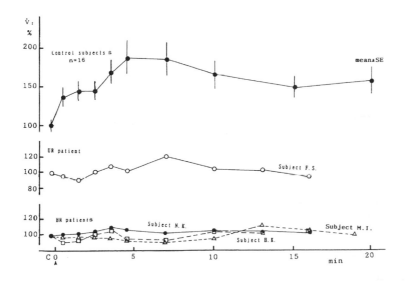

Figure 2. Comparison of time couse of hypoxic ventilatory responses among the control subjects and UR nd BR patients in terms of relative % magnitude to that in the control period. Both control subjects and the UR patient revealed Biph. HVD, whereas the BR patients exhibited a completely different profile.

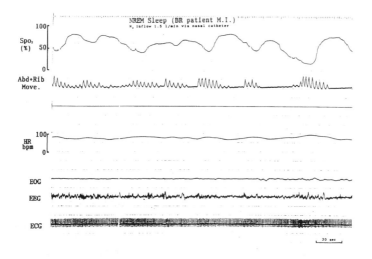

Figure 3. Respiratory response to N_2 gas administration into the nasal cavity at a flow rate of 1.5 l/min during slow wave non-REM sleep in BR subject M.I. Arterial desaturation was advanced as low as less than SPO_2 50% with repetition of apneic episodes.

Discussion

In contrast to the control subjects and UR patient, all three BR patients lost the specific Biph.HVD profile during sustained hypoxic exposure. In addition, their V_I in the late hypoxic period was not depressed to less than the pre-hypoxic level as was seen in UR patient. These results were considered to indicate that the CB plays indispensable roles in eliciting HVD.

Although observation of ventilatory response to sustained hypoxia in BR patients has only been made by us, Dahan et al. recently obtained similar findings in human volunteers whose V_I was kept inhibited at pre-hypoxic levels by the continuous infusion of dopamine.[12] Thus, it seems certain in humans that the loss of initial hypoxic hyperventilation is inevitably not accompanied by HVD. Loss of Biph.HVD in two BR patients was already reported by us.[14-18] In this paper, we further obtained one more BR patient and supplemented sleep studies with hypoxia. Thus, taking into consideration all the data accumulated, we have developed a new concept for the function of CB.

We have also noted that the ventilatory level in the BRs showed the tendency to slightly increase in the late period of hypoxia. During moderate to intense hypoxia, occurrence of gradual hyperventilation has long been recognized even after the carotid sinus nerve sectioning in awake cats,[19,20] dogs,[21,22] and rabbits,[22] or in goats,[23,24] whose carotid body was separately perfused by euoxemic blood during systemic hypoxia. By ablation studies and other observations on ventilatory variables, the site of its neuronal origin was inferred to be located in the so-called defense area in the diencephalon.[25-29] Granted that the slight hyperpnea in response to mild hypoxia observed BR patients is of the same nature as that centrally originating hyperventilation reported in above animal studies, the loss of secondary hypoxic decline may be explained by a lack of afferent information from the CB to the above diencephalic area via the solitary tract nuclei (NTS). The lack of HVD in BR patients was in marked contrast to that reported in anesthetized with CB-denervated animals which exhibited long-lasting hypoxic ventilatory depression to less than pre-hypoxic level during and even after hypoxic exposure.[30,31] This difference between awake and anesthetized animals may be explained by the strong depressant influence of anesthesia or narcotics on the diencephalic area responsible for centrally originating hypoxic hyperventilation. To examine a similar influence for depressing consciousness on V_I, we further studied two BR patients. Simple whole night follow up exhibited no particular disturbances. However, when N_2 gas was administered during non-rapid eye movement (non-REM) in patient M.I. and sleep stage was advanced to slow wave state, severe desaturation as low as around SPO_2 50% developed during this period with repetition of apneic episodes (Fig. 3). In contrast, no such SPO_2 fall was seen during rapid eye movement (REM) sleep with corticobulbal activation. It was noted that during REM sleep patients took a lateral sleeping position which is known as a characteristic behavioral movement in this sleep stage, and it was considered that such a posture was effective in preventing the development of airway obstruction and arterial desaturation. It was further postulated that the diencephalic area is activated during REM sleep and is concerned with inducing this behavioral activity.

Taking into consideration the present results and the information available in the literatures, we constructed a schema to explain a possible mechanism for the Biph.HVD in mild hypoxia in awake humans (Fig. 4). The concerned organ and areas are the CB and its afferent input station, NTS, in the medulla, brainstem respiratory center complex (RC), the diencephalic area (DA) and the cortical area (CA). The neuronal reciprocal innervation connecting these structures are well documented in the literature.[28] Since CB denervation during hypoxia in the awake state resulted in the loss of both initial hyperpnea and secondary HVD and may have disclosed DA-originating gradual hyperventilation during late period of sustained hypoxia, there must have existed an inhibitory information to induce HVD from NTS to DA before carotid chemodenervation. The most plausible experimental evidence to explain this inhibition at present appears to be dopamine release with time in the NTS as reported by Goiny et al.[32] However, it must be emphasized that dopamine hypothesis for HVD is still a matter of considerable controversy.[33,34] With anesthesia, narcotics or induced deep sleep, DA may be strongly inhibited and ventilatory depression will be sustained. Depressed cortical inhibition or facilitation on DA may also be induced, depending on the state of non-REM or REM sleep. The major difference in Biph.HVD between anesthetized animals and awake humans may stem from this mechanism, as discussed by Robbins.[8]

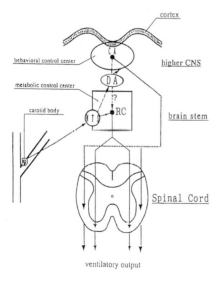

Figure 4. Possible mechanism to explain biphasic hypoxic ventilatory decline (Biph.HVD) in awake humans. CA: cortical area, DA: diencephalic area, CB: carotid body, NTS: solitary tract nucleus, RC: Brainstem respiratory center complex. Solid line and broken line indicate stimulation and inhibition, respectively. Inhibition from NTS to DA, or possibly to RC, increases with time, so Biph.HVD will be developed during sustained hypoxic exposure. DA is susceptible to anesthesia, narcotics and deep sleep, and is depressed with the induction of hypoventilation and desaturation. The solid line from the RC and the chain line from the behavioral control center are the ventilatory output pathways for metabolic and behavioral respiratory control, respectively.

In recent years, evidence has been accumulating that HVD in mild hypoxia is a useful adaptation for living organisms.[7] It economizes energy expenditure and stabilizes cellular activity of the nervous and respiratory systems due to induced membrane hyperpolarization.

Yet, brain cellular energy charges as evaluated by the concentrations of high energy phosphate compounds and of lactate are well preserved.[35] Maximal respiratory responses to hypercapnia and hypoxia are still well maintained, indicating that the metabolic control capacity of the respiratory system is not essentially impaired.[36-38] The facts that, in normal subjects, this useful HVD is linearly correlated with the initial hypoxic hyperventilation (Fig. 1) and the BR subjects lost specific Biph. HVD pattern, led us to assume that initial CB excitation may, in some way, induce the subsequent HVD in proportional amount.

Finally, it may be argued that chemosensitivity of the BR patients may have modified by neuronal plasticity change during long period after surgery. Although recovery of peripheral chemosensitivity was reported in cats and in ponies,[39,40] our previous data indicated that this is unlikely in humans[15,41]

In conclusion, we now propose that CB not only is important for preventing further advancing of hypoxemia by eliciting hyperventilation but also plays a useful role in controlling the degree of subsequent ventilatory decline within the range of mild hypoxia.

We are grateful for Prof. A. Guz for his useful suggestion for conducting the sleep study in hypoxia.

References

1. Heymans C, Bouckhaert JJ, Dautrebande L. Sinus carotidien et reflexes respiratoires II. Influences respiratoires reflexes de l'acidose, de l'alcalose, de l'anhydride carbonique, de l'ion hydrogene et de l'anoxeme. Sinus carotidiens et echanges respiratores dans les poumons et au dela des poumons. *Arch Internat Pharmaocodyn* 39: 400-448, 1930.
2. Weil JV, Zwillich CW. Assessment of ventilatory response to hypoxia. Method and interpretation. *Chest* 70 (Suppl.): 124-128, 1976.
3. Easton PA, Slykerman LT, Anthonisen NR. Ventilatory response to sustained hypoxia in normal adults. *J Appl Physiol* 61: 906-911, 1986.
4. Khamnei S, Robbins PA. Hypoxic depression of ventilation in humans: alternative models for the chemoreflexes. *Respir Physiol* 81: 117-134, 1990.
5. Vizek M, Pickett CK, Weil JV. Biphasic ventilatory response of adult cats to sustained hypoxia has central origin. *J Appl Physiol* 63: 1658-1664, 1987.
6. Bascom DA, Clement ID, Cunningham DA, Painter R, Robbins PA. Changes in peripheral chemoreflex sensitivity during sustained, isocapnic hypoxia. *Respir Physiol* 82: 161-176, 1990.
7. Neubauer JA, Melton JE, Edelman NH. Modulation of respiration during brain hypoxia. *J Appl Physiol* 68: 441-451, 1990.
8. Robbins PA. Hypoxic ventilatory decline: site of action. *J Appl Physiol* 79: 373-374, 1995.
9. Honda Y. Ventilatory depression during mild hypoxia in adult humans. *Jpn J Physiol* 45: 947-959, 1995.
10. Bureau MA, Zinman R. Foulon P, Begin R. Diphasic ventilatory response to hypoxia in newborn lambs. *J Appl Physiol* 56: 84-90, 1984.
11. Georgopoulos D, Walker S, Anthonisen NR. Increased chemoreceptor output and ventilatory response to sustained hypoxia. *J Appl Physiol* 67: 1157-1163, 1989.
12. Dahan A. Ward D, van den Elsen M, Temp J, Berkenbosch A. Influence of reduced carotid body drive during sustained hypoxia on hypoxic depression of ventilation in humans. *J Appl Physiol* 81: 565-572, 1996.
13. Honda Y, Tani H, Masuda A, Kobayashi T, Nishino T, Kimura H, Masuyama S, Kuriyama

T. Effect of prior O_2 breathing on ventilatory response to sustained isocapnic hypoxia in awake humans. *J Appl Physiol* 81: 1627-1632, 1996.

14. Tanaka M, Kimura H, Kunitomo F, Sakuma T, Kurono T, Hasako K, Uruma T, Kuriyama T, Honda Y. Effect of sustained hypoxia on ventilatory and heart rate responses in carotid body-resected humans. *Jpn J Appl Physiol* 22: 81-87, 1992.

15. Honda Y.Respiratory and circulatory activities in carotid body-resected humans. *J Appl Physiol* 73: 1-8, 1992.

16. Honda Y, Tanaka M. Respiratory and cardiovascular activities in carotid body-resected humans. In: *Neurobiology and Cell Physiology of Chemoreception*. Edited by Data PG, Acker H, Lahiri S. New York, Plenum Press, pp 359-364, 1993.

17. Honda Y. Dual functions of the carotid body: a hypothesis based on observations in patients with its resection. *J Physiol Lond* 497: 26p-27p, 1996.

18. Honda Y, Kimura H, Tanaka M. Role of carotid body activity responsible for hypoxic ventilatory decline in awake humans. *J Appl Physiol* 82: 37, 1997.

19. Miller MJ, Tenney SM. Hypoxia-induced tachypnea in carotid-deafferented cats. *Respir Physiol* 23: 31-39, 1975.

20. Gautier H, Bonora M. Effect of carotid body denervation on respiratory pattern of adult cats. *J Appl Physiol* 46: 1127-1131, 1979.

21. Davenport HW, Brewer G, Chambers AH, Goldschmidt S. The respiratory responses to anoxemia of unanesthetized dogs with chronically denervated aortic and carotid chemoreceptors and their causes. *Am J Physiol* 148: 406-416, 1947.

22. Bouverot P, Candas U, Libert JP. Role of the arterial chemoreceptors in ventilatory adaptation to hypoxia of awake dogs and rabbits. *Respir Physiol* 17: 209-219, 1973.

23. Weizhen N, Engwall MJA, Daristotle L, Pizarro J, Bisgard GE. Ventilatory effects of prolonged systemic (CNS) hypoxia in awake goats. *Respir Physiol* 87: 37-48, 1992.

24. Smith CA, Engwall MJA, Dempsey JA, Bisgard GE. Effects of specific carotid body and brain hypoxia on respiratory muscle control in the awake goat. *J Physiol Lond* 460: 623-640, 1993.

25. Hilton SM. The defence-arousal system and its relevance for circulatory and respiratory control. *J Exp Biol* 100: 159-174, 1982.

26. Tenney SM, Ou LC. Ventilatory response of decorticate and decerebrate cats to hypoxia and CO_2. *Respir Physiol* 29: 81-92, 1977.

27. Nielsen AM, Bisgard GE,. Mitchell GS. Phrenic nerve responses to hypoxia and CO_2 in decerebrate dogs. *Respir Physiol* 65: 267-283, 1986.

28. Waldrop TG, Porter JP. Hypothalamic involvement in respiratory and cardiovascular regulation. In: *Regulation of Breathing. 2nd edition*. Edited by Dempsey JA, Pack.AI. New York, Marcel Dekker Inc, pp 315-364, 1995.

29. Bisgard GE, Neubauer JA. Peripheral and central effect of hypoxia. In: *Regulation of Breathing. 2nd edition*. Edited by Dempsey JA, Pack AI. New York, Marcel Dekker Inc, pp 617-667, 1995.

30. Bouckhaert JJ. Heymans C, Samaan A. The role of carotid sinus and vagal chemoreceptors in the respiratory and vasomotor effects of hypoxaemia in anaesthetized and normal dogs. *J Physiol Lond* 94: 4p-5p, 1938.

31. Millhorn DE, Eldridge FL, Kiley JP, Waldrop TG. Prolonged inhibition of respiration following acute hypoxia on glomectomized cats. *Respir Physiol* 57: 331-340, 1984.

32. Goiny H, Lagercrantz H, Srinivasan M, Ungerstedt U, Yamamoto Y. Hypoxia-mediated in vivo release of dopamine in nucleus tractus solitarii of rabbits. *J Appl Physiol* 70: 2395-2400, 1991.

33. Tatsumi K, Pickett CK, Weil JV. Effects of haloperidol and domperidone on ventilatory roll

off during sustained hypoxia in cats. *J Appl Physiol* 72: 1945-1952, 1992

34. Pedersen MEF, Dorrington KL, Robbins PA. Effect of haloperidol on ventilation during isocapnic hypoxia in humans. *J Appl Physiol* 83: 1110-1115, 1997.
35. Siejö BK, Nilsson L. The influence of arterial hypoxemia upon labile phosphates and upon extracellular lactate and pyruvate concentration in the rat brain. *Scand J Lab Clin Invest* 27: 83-96, 1971.
36. Melton JE, Neubauer JA, Edelman NH. CO_2 sensitivity of cat phrenic neurogram during hypoxic respiratory depression. *J Appl Physiol* 65: 736-743, 1988.
37. Melton,JE, Chae LO, Neubauer JA, Edelman NH. Extracellular potassium homeostasis in the cat medulla during progressive brain hypoxia. *J Appl Physiol* 70: 1477-1482, 1991.
38. Neubauer JA, Melton JE, Yu Q, Chae LO, Edelman NH. Modulation of respiration by brain hypoxia. In: *Control of breathing and its modeling perspective.* Edited by Honda Y, Miyamoto Y, Konno K, Widdicombe JG. New York, Plenum Press, pp 307-310, 1992.
39. Smith PG, Mills E. Restoration of reflex ventilatory response to hypoxia after removal of carotid bodies in the cat. *Neurosci* 5: 573-580, 1980.
40. Bisgard GE, Forster HV, Klein JP. Recovery of peripheral chemoreceptor function after denervation in ponies. *J Appl Physiol (Respir Environ Exercise Physiol)* 48: 964-970, 1980.
41. Honda Y. Ventilatory activities in humans vs some other mammals after carotid body resection. *Funktionsanalyse biologischer Systeme.* 23: 313-317, 1993.

Effects of hypoxia and hypercapnia on cardiac contractility and energetics

Johannes H.G.M. van Beek

The main goal of the regulation of lung ventilation is to maintain blood concentrations of oxygen and carbon dioxide at physiological levels.[1] Here we will consider effects of hypoxia and hypercapnia on the heart, the pump which takes care of the transport of oxygen and carbon dioxide between the lung and the rest of the body. Oxygen supply to the heart tissue is essential to provide energy for the cardiac pump function. Depression of cardiac aerobic metabolism is dangerous, because the heart provides the driving force for its own perfusion and oxygen supply. A surplus of carbon dioxide in the blood, hypercapnia, leads to a fast increase in acidity in the heart muscle cell, suppressing cardiac contractility. Adequate control of lung ventilation is therefore important to the heart, but we will see that the heart itself can cope with hypoxemia and hypercapnia within certain limits.

Hypoxia and the heart

If blood oxygen concentration falls, usually the arterial blood pressure rises, because of peripheral vasoconstriction brought about by stimulation of the chemoreflexes.[2] This is often accompanied by slowing of the heart rate. Such increases in blood pressure caused by hypoxemia may increase the work load on the heart, but bradycardia limits this increase. If the high blood pressure caused by hypoxemia recurs often, this might lead to cardiac hypertrophy. At the same time that the cardiac work load is increased somewhat, the oxygen supply to cardiac tissue is decreased. Progressive hypoxemia depresses cardiac contractility (i.e., the cardiac contractile force under fixed loading conditions). Although a statistically significant depression of cardiac contractility by half was found only at an arterial oxygen saturation of 63% in anesthetized dogs, it is likely that there is a gradual mild depression of cardiac contractility as arterial oxygen saturation drops below the baseline value of 94%.[3] In the intact organism, the direct effect of hypoxemia on cardiac metabolism and work may be counteracted by regulatory mechanisms, neural and hormonal, and by peripheral vasoregulation. If hypoxic depression of cardiac metabolism decreases cardiac contractility, the sympathetic nerves might partially compensate by stimulating the heart muscle.

To see the direct effect of hypoxia on the heart muscle we examine what happens in isolated perfused hearts which are not influenced by regulatory influences coming from the rest of the body. The contractile force of the heart declines when oxygen is almost totally removed from the perfusate of the heart, but it is remarkable that the heart keeps beating for a long time (at least 15 min) with no oxygen present, as long as the heart is still perfused and anaerobic glycolysis is possible, see figure 1. However, when perfusion of the heart is stopped, cardiac contractility declines rapidly to zero within five minutes.[4] When glycolysis is prevented during high-flow anoxia, the cardiac developed pressure declines rapidly, as in no-flow ischemia.[5] If the arterial oxygen tension in a saline perfusate is gradually decreased, while maintaining the coronary flow during extracorporeal perfusion, cardiac contractile performance was found to be maintained until oxygen tension is decreased from ~600 mmHg to below ~200 mmHg.[6] However, in the same isolated hearts cardiac oxygen consumption decreases often even for small decreases in arterial oxygen tension on the order of 10-20%.[6,7] It is remarkable that for anesthetized dogs an increase in cardiac oxygen consumption has been reported during mild hypoxemia, even when changes in heart rate and cardiac output were controlled.[8]

The coronary vessels dilate in response to arterial hypoxemia, and the increased coronary flow compensates for decreased blood oxygen content.[9] In some patients inhaling 100% oxygen, the myocardial blood flow falls, and myocardial oxygen availability may not increase.[10] As is the case for the regulation of lung ventilation, increased carbon dioxide tension potentiates the increase of coronary blood flow caused by hypoxia.

Increases in glycolysis, coronary blood flow and oxygen extraction are three mechanisms by which the heart may counteract the hypoxic depression of myocardial aerobic metabolism. Oxygen consumption is not much depressed and cardiac output is still reasonably well maintained until arterial oxygen saturation falls below 70%.[3] However, for severe reductions in arterial oxygen saturation depression of myocardial metabolism does lead to severe limitation of cardiac contractility.

The heart after reoxygenation

Reintroduction of oxygen into the heart after a brief period of ischemia or anoxia does alleviate the immediate problems of tissue hypoxia, but can introduce new problems due to reperfusion/reoxygenation damage by generation of reactive oxygen species, which cause the contractility of the heart to be depressed for many days. A brief period of ischemia (for instance <20 min) does not yet lead to irreversible tissue damage, as longer oxygen deprivation would. However, cardiac contractility can still be decreased for a long time, despite the reoxygenation, a condition known as myocardial stunning (see fig. 1). Many causes have been proposed for myocardial stunning, for instance damage to excitation-contraction coupling, contractile machinery, collagen, etc. However, the mitochondria appeared to be remarkably resistant to damage and disturbances of energy supply to the myofibrils were not thought to be the cause of myocardial stunning.[4]

ATP is hydrolyzed during cardiac contraction at the cross bridges in the myofibrils and at the ion pumps. The main site of ATP synthesis is at the mitochondria. We have proposed that the energetic signal may travel slowly through the myoplasm between sites of ATP hydrolysis and aerobic ATP synthesis. We have developed methods to assess the speed of the response of myocardial oxidative phosphorylation to steps in cardiac workload, using fast responding oxygen electrodes and mathematical model calculations to correct for diffusion and intravascular transport delays,[11] and to simultaneously measure the time course of changes of phosphocreatine and inorganic phosphate using ^{31}P-NMR spectroscopy.[12] Using these methods we found that phosphocreatine (PCr) is broken down quickly when heart rate and thereby ATP hydrolysis rate are increased. PCr is used for resynthesis of ATP

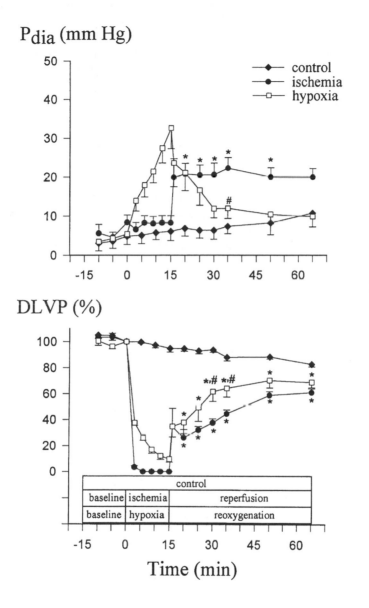

Figure 1. Cardiac contractile function during and after hypoxia and ischemia. The end-diastolic pressure (Pdia) and the developed left ventricular pressure (DLVP) in isolated saline-perfused rabbit hearts at 37 °C is plotted during and after 15 min high-flow hypoxia (oxygen tension 19 mmHg) or ischemia starting at t=0. DLVP (systolic minus diastolic pressure) is set to 100% at t=0. Mean ± SEM. Paced heart rate 100 beats/min. Some error bars fall within symbols. * $P<0.05$ vs. control; # $P<0.05$ hypoxia vs ischemia. [From: ref. 4. Permission was granted by Waverly].

in the reaction catalyzed by creatine kinase. PCr decreases with a time constant on the order of 3 s, and the inorganic phosphate, which results from the breakdown of ATP, increased with a time course mirroring the decrease in PCr. However, the increase in oxidative phosphorylation was much slower, with time constant 11 s in the same experiment.[11,12] We have proposed that the energetic signal necessary to stimulate oxidative phosphorylation in the mitochondria is related to the phosphate metabolites which change quickly, but that these phosphate metabolites do initially change only in or near the myofibrils and ion pumps and do then reach the mitochondria with a delay of several seconds, causing delay in the stimulation of the mitochondria.[13] This would mean that transfer of energy through the myofibrils, across the cytosol and the mitochondrial outer membrane is slow and may therefore not occur by simple free diffusion of phosphate metabolites, but may depend on the structural integrity of the cell.

We found in isolated rabbit hearts that after myocardial stunning the response time of oxygen consumption to heart rate steps increased by ~40%.[4] After brief ischemia or hypoxia oxidative phosphorylation therefore responded slower to heart rate steps, despite the reoxygenation. We proposed that energy transfer or signaling between sites of ATP hydrolysis and oxidative phosphorylation is affected in stunned myocardium, and may contribute to the contractile dysfunction after brief ischemia.

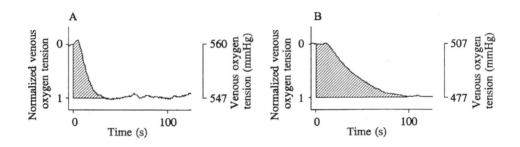

Figure 2. Effect of hypercapnia on the response of cardiac oxygen consumption to heart rate steps. Cardiac oxygen consumption increases linearly with the decrease in coronary venous oxygen tension, because perfusion flow is kept constant. At t=0 the paced heart rate is suddenly increased. The perfusate was gassed with 5% CO2 (panel A) or 23% CO_2 (panel B). The perfusate pH was 7.3 and 6.6 respectively. The experiment was done on isolated rabbit heart at 28 °C. The measured venous response time, obtained by integrating the hatched area after normalization to 0 at start and 1 at end of response, was 19 s in panel A and 35 s in panel B. These venous response times are corrected for the time taken by diffusion and intravascular transport to obtain the response time at the level of the mitochondria, see text. [From; ref. 17. Permission was granted by Springer-Verlag].

However, the effect of very brief ischemia, shorter than the 15 min of flow interruption leading to stunning, may not be deleterious, but may even be protective to the heart. A period of long ischemia may lead to less tissue damage and fewer cardiac arrhythmias if it is preceded by a short period of ischemia followed by reperfusion. This phenomenon is termed cardiac preconditioning.

Hypercapnia and the heart

When carbon dioxide tension increases and/or pH decreases in the coronary perfusate, the contractility of the heart is depressed because the intracellular pH decreases. On the other hand, when the perfusate becomes more alkaline, cardiac contractility is increased above control levels. Intracellular acidosis also occurs when flow is stopped or decreased. During acute respiratory acidosis, cardiac contractility is strongly depressed at first, but then recovers partially because the intracellular pH recovers at unchanged CO_2 tension mediated via Na^+-H^+ exchange.[14]

Intracellular acidosis affects many steps in the excitation-contraction pathway.[15] Both the release of Ca^{2+} into the cytosol which is the trigger for cardiac contraction and the sensitivity of the contractile proteins to Ca^{2+} are decreased. However, the maximal oxygen consumption of isolated cardiac mitochondria is only decreased by 10-15% if the pH of the medium is brought down from 7.1 to 6.5, a value that is found in the cytosol during cardiac ischemia.[16] This reduction of oxidative phosphorylation was similar whether brought about by high concentrations of carbon dioxide, or with metabolic acidosis. Apparently, the energetic status of the heart is not much deteriorated by mild acidosis,[15] and ATP and PCr levels are not drastically altered, so that mitochondrial ATP production does not appear to be a limiting factor under these conditions. Severe acidosis inhibits the glycolytic chain at the level of phosphofructokinase and inhibits the Krebs cycle at the level of citrate synthase, hindering both anaerobic and aerobic ATP synthesis.

The transfer time for the energetic signal through the cell becomes much slower during intracellular acidosis brought about by hypercapnia, see figure 2. In isolated rabbit hearts tested at 28 °C the response time of mitochondrial oxygen consumption to heart rate steps increased from 14.4 s to 22-36 s due to acidosis, depending on the time at which acidosis is applied.[17] Here the CO_2 level for gassing the perfusate was increased from 5 to 23%, changing the intracellular pH from 7.1 to 6.5. In contrast to what happens upon reoxygenation after hypoxia, the effect of hypercapnia on the response time of oxygen consumption is completely reversible. Because it appears that the mitochondrial capacity for oxidative phosphorylation is not much diminished, we hypothesize that the increase of the response time of oxygen consumption means that the transfer of energy through the cytosol is slowed. This might contribute to the decreased contractility during hypercapnia, despite the fact that the mitochondria themselves are not much inhibited.

Summary

The heart has compensatory mechanisms for mild hypoxemia and hypercapnia, but severe hypoxemia and hypercapnia may depress cardiac contractility strongly. We propose that impaired transfer of high-energy phosphate groups through the heart muscle cell, caused by hypercapnia or by hypoxia followed by reoxygenation, may contribute to the decreased cardiac contractility found during hypercapnia or during myocardial stunning.

Acknowledgment: J van Beek is an established investigator of the Netherlands Heart Foundation.

References
1. Berkenbosch A. *Chemical Control of Breathing*. Thesis, Rijksuniversiteit Leiden, 1987.
2. Van den Aardweg JG. *Cardiovascular Effects of Cyclic Changes in Breathing Pattern*. Thesis, Universiteit van Amsterdam, 1992.
3. Walley KR, Becker CJ, Hogan RA, Teplinsky K, Wood LDH. Progressive hypoxemia limits left ventricular oxygen consumption and contractility. *Circ Res* 63:849-859, 1988.
4. Zuurbier CJ, van Beek JHGM. Mitochondrial response to heart rate steps in isolated rabbit heart is slowed after myocardial stunning. *Circ Res* 81:69-75, 1997.
5. Allen DG, Orchard CH. Myocardial contractile function during ischemia and hypoxia. *Circ Res* 60:153-168, 1987.
6. Ito K, Nioka S, Chance B. Oxygen dependence of energy state and cardiac work in the perfused rat heart. In: J. Piiper ed. *Oxygen Transport to Tissue XII*. Plenum, New York, pp. 449-457, 1990.
7. Van Beek JHGM, Bouma P, Westerhof N. Oxygen uptake in saline-perfused rabbit heart is decreased to a similar extent during reductions in flow and in arterial oxygen concentration. *Pflügers Arch (Eur J Physiol)* 414: 82-88, 1989.
8. Powers ER, Powell WJ. Effect of arterial hypoxia on myocardial oxygen consumption. *Circ Res* 33: 749-756, 1973.
9. Broten TP, Romson JL, Fullerton AD, Van Winkle DM, Feigl EO. Synergistic action of myocardial oxygen and carbon dioxide in controlling coronary blood flow. *Circ Res* 68:531-542, 1991.
10. Kenmure ACF, Beatson JMcD, Cameron AJV, Horton PW. Effect of oxygen on myocardial blood flow and metabolism. *Cardiovasc Res* 5:483-489, 1971.
11. Van Beek JHGM, Westerhof N. Response time of cardiac mitochondrial oxygen consumption to heart rate steps. *Am J Physiol* 260:H613-H625, 1991.
12. Eijgelshoven MHJ, van Beek JHGM, Mottet I, Nederhoff MGJ, van Echteld CJA, Westerhof N. Cardiac high-energy phosphates adapt faster than oxygen consumption to changes in heart rate.*Circ Res* 75: 751-759, 1994.
13. Van Beek JHGM, Tian X, Zuurbier CJ, de Groot B, van Echteld CJA, Eijgelshoven MHJ, Hak JB. The dynamic regulation of myocardial oxidative phosphorylation. Analysis of the response time of oxygen consumption (Review). *Moll Cell Biochem*, in press.
14. Cingolani HE, Koretsune Y, Marban E. Recovery of contractility and pH_i during respiratory acidosis in ferret hearts: role of Na^+-H^+ exchange. *Am J Physiol* 259: H843-H848, 1990.
15. Orchard CH, Kentish JC. Effects of changes of pH on the contractile function of heart muscle. *Am J Physiol* 258: C967-C981, 1990.
16. Van Wijhe MH, Van Beek JHGM. Effects of respiratory and metabolic acidosis on oxidative phosphorylation in isolated rabbit heart mitochondria. *Pflügers Arch. (Eur J Physiol)* 430: R174, 1995.
17. Hak JB, van Beek JHGM, Westerhof N. Acidosis slows the response of oxidative phosphorylation to metabolic demand in isolated rabbit heart. *Pflügers Arch (Europ J Physiol)* 423: 324-329, 1993.

Tissue oxygenation-monitoring using Near Infra Red Spectroscopy

Berend Oeseburg

Introduction

The supply and distribution of oxygen in tissues is extremely heterogeneous in various types of tissue as was already shown in the sixties by the application of micro-pO_2 electrodes to monitor the distribution of pO_2 throughout tissues like brain, liver, myocardium and muscle. High pO_2's at the arterial side of a capillary network, low pO_2's in between the capillaries. Although this invasive and time-consuming technique has been applied in clinical situations it never became a routine method for the monitoring of tissue oxygenation.

The introduction of Near InfraRed Spectroscopy (NIRS)[2,3,4,7,16,20] seemed a promising concept since it provided us with a non invasive, continuous and easily applicable optical system for the monitoring of oxyhemoglobin and de-oxyhemoglobin in various tissues. These signals of course are directly related to the oxygenation of the tissue of interest. A few 'minor' problems remain: like the unknown pathlength of the photons,[12,25] the unknown scattering of the photons and the unknown influence of absorption in the superficial layers, above the region of interest. This makes that still only qualitative (but striking!) instead of quantitative information is made available with NIRS systems. One special problem only recently recognised in the 'NIRS world' is the fact that we do not know the source of signals. How much information on oxyhemoglobin and de-oxyhemoglobin is from larger vessels?, arteries? as well as veins?, all capillaries? or just a few? The only way to get informed about these uncertainties is to (re-)apply the modelling of tissue compartments similar to the evaluation of the micro-pO_2 histograms from the sixties.

Methods

Near infrared spectroscopy makes use of the facts that biological tissues are relative transparent for light in the infrared region and that the absorption of that light is dependent to the redox state of cytochrome and the oxygenation state of haemoglobin in the trans-illuminated area as first described by Jöbsis van der Vliet. The method is based on sequential pulsing a number (3 minimal) of lasers in the near infra red region and sending this light into tissue through the skin using optical fibres. The penetrated light scatters and some of the scattered light can be picked up by an other optical fibre either coupled to a photomultiplier tube (PMT) or a photoavalance diode (PAD). By coupling sending and receiving algorithms the discrimination of the received pulses to their initial wavelengths is easy. The observed changes in optical density at each wavelength then are converted to relative changes in the concentrations of the oxygen dependent chromophores. This conversion is simply based on Lambert-Beers law by introducing the known extinction coefficients of the components of interest and an assumed differential pathlength factor (DPF). The latter is obtained from a number of experiments on preferably the same tissue using a time of flight (TOF) measuring system. World wide only a few TOF systems are available due to the very high costs (± 1 Million US $) and the limited applicability due to the complex set-up. This makes that the obtained signals are always rough estimates of the absolute concentrations and that is why nearly all groups report relative changes in the concentrations of the oxygen dependent chromophores only. These signals, however, provide continuous information on the oxygenation of the tissue of interest and thus can be used as a reliable trend monitor at least. Furthermore, by applying external interventions to the gas exchange, the local circulation, posture, cortical stimuly or medication; NIRS signals can be used in these situations to calculate local blood volume, local oxygen consumption, active blood volume and local adaptations in oxygenation due to the intervention.

Results
Since a limited space is available and most of the results are already presented in international journals. Therefore an substantial volume of the space available is used for references. Only a few examples of our results in a variety of applications, clinical as well as fundamental, will be worked out briefly.

Cerebral oxygenation in Neonatology [13,2,7]
This is the field covered by most NIRS users since the neonatal skull and brain are relative transparent for NIR light. Liem[24] did describe 2 striking findings in his applications. In the first series he followed the cerebral oxygenation of neonates treated with indomethacine. This drug is applied to those neonates who show no spontaneous closure of the ductus arteriosus, a connection between the pulmonary artery and aorta, which closes normally within 24 hours after birth. If not, indomethacine induces closure after application within the next 24 hours. By monitoring the cerebral oxygenation using NIRS[22] he found in all patients an tremendous decrease in oxygenation both with a bolus injection or a slow infusion of the same amount of indomethacine. Therefore he concluded that only babies without anaemia and normal arterial blood gases could be treated without risk. Moreover, these findings initiated the search for a better drug for this treatment. This is the first report where NIRS measurements resulted in the change in clinical treatment.

A number of newborns suffer from respiratory problems in such a degree that the survival rate is < 80% on conventional treatment. In these cases the ultimate treatment is extra corporeal membrane oxygenation (ECMO); a technique that takes over both heart and lung function using a heart lung machine for 24 h - 4 wk. Venous blood is drained from the right atrium by a canula introduced into the right jugular vein and, after oxygenation, re-introduced into the aorta by a canula introduced into the right common carotid artery. These occlusive canulae completely block the supply and drain through artery and vein respectively. By applying NIRS[23] we could prove that the common idea of a decreased oxygenation of the right half of the brain was not available and so we could objectively prove the safety of this canulation.

Cerebral oxygenation in Adults [9,10,14]

In his more basic research to find out "if NIRS is a toy or a tool?" Colier did a number a experiments including the influence of posture changes on cerebral oxygenation in volunteers.[7] One of the volunteers showed an abnormal reaction in the NIRS tracing preceding an episode of spontaneous fainting due to, what seemed, ortho-static hypotension.[8,17,18,19] We could repeat this with this volunteer but none of the others ever showed such an episode. The protocol was repeated with 16 volunteers before and directly after the donation of 0.5 L whole blood to the local blood bank. To show the relation between NIRS tracing and ortho-static hypotension all volunteers were hooked up with a noninvasive blood pressure measuring system (Finapres®). The results are collected in Table 1.

Table 1. The rate of change (slope) of oxygenation index (OI) and blood volume (tHb) in the head-up position, before and after withdrawal of blood. After withdrawal a significant difference (* $p = 0.02$) in OI is found between the fainters (n = 6) and the non-fainters (n = 4). No significant differences were found for the tHb signal.

	Before withdrawal		After withdrawal	
	Fainter	**Non-fainter**	**Fainter**	**Non-fainter**
Slope tHb	0.15 ± 0.13	0.08 ± 0.08	0.03 ± 0.45	0.19 ± 0.33
Slope OI	-0.06 ± 0.18	-0.16 ± 0.31	-1.4 ± 1.4 *	-0.18 ± 0.33
Slope OI (during presyncope)	NA	NA	-5.2 ± 4.2	NA

Units μM·min^{-1} (mean ± SD); NA not applicable

The signals are visualised in Figure 1 from which it is clear that the continuous fall in cerebral oxygenation in the fainters show a great mismatch between oxygen supply and oxygen demand in the brain. This continuous mismatch induces, later on, the hypotension. Thus the 'common knowledge': orthostatic hypotension induces cerebral dysoxygenation is not supported by this finding. It is the other way around!

Oxygenation in other tissues

In Urology a number of protocols are used for the surgery on cryptorchism;[1,6] a situation where the testis is not descended into the scrotum. In most of these protocols a number of supplying blood vessels have to be ligated and cut, resulting in a badly perfused testis until revascularisation takes place. In the clinical situation it is impossible to predict if the used protocol leads to a cosmetic result only or also to functional testis. Therefore the protocols where applied in animal experiments with NIRS for the measurement of the so called active

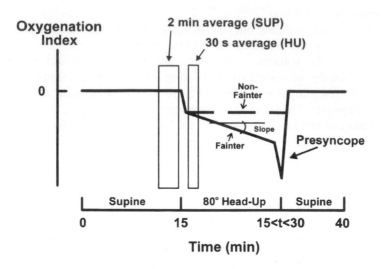

Figure 1. A schematic representation of the time course of the experiment and the analysis performed on the signals. After 15 min in supine (SUP) position the subject is tilted to an 80° head-up position (HU) for 15 min. or less if the subject faints. The experiment ends with a 10 period in supine position. For clarity only the oxygenation index (OI), being the difference of oxy- and deoxyhaemoglobin, is displayed.

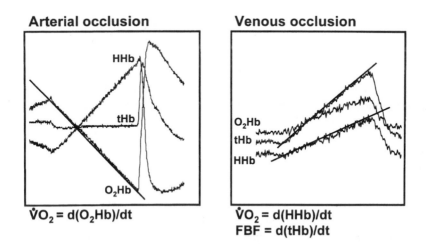

Figure 2. NIRS tracing during arterial occlusion (left panel) and venous occlusion (right panel). From the various slopes oxygen consumption, blood volume and blood flow can be calculated.

blood volume (ABV), defined as the fraction of the blood still actively circulating after clamping of one of the supplying arteries. The operations were finished lege artis where in half of the animals the procedure resulting in a low to absent ABV was used and in the other half the procedure with a high ATB. Three month afterwards autopsy proved that all testis with a low ABT were atrophic while all testis with a high ATB proved normal. These striking results will sooner or later lead to an adapted NIRS system suitable for use during the clinical operations.

Neurologists are confronted with patients with complaints of chronic fatigue, diagnosis of it being complicated, costly, time consuming and invasive. A substantial part of this group of patients prove to muscular disease with abnormal mitochondrial function. Theoretical this must be displayed by an abnormal oxygen consumption during contraction. Up till now this can only be quantified by in invasive test to obtain blood samples from the muscle region of interest for analysis of metabolites. Applying NIRS to these muscles[5,11,15,21] enables us to calculate oxygen consumption, local blood volume and blood flow as is shown in Figure 2.

Due to the unknown DPF in this application we are just in the basic test phase of this project in which we try to find a modulating factor, based on skinfold measurements, for the individual adjustment of the DPF.

Discussion

From the presented examples as well as from references it becomes clear that NIRS is a potential tool in the assessment of tissue oxygenation, provided that the interpretation of the results is done carefully and with full knowledge of the limitations. There are numerous papers, I apologize beforehand, mainly from clinical groups without support of basic scientist, in which conclusions are presented that can not be repeated by others. We are aware even of publications, not in the list below, where tracings obtain on different days after removing and reapplication of the probes are treated as one 'continuous' registrations. In their discussion they certainly were not aware of changes in DPF, measured area or even changes in distant between optodes and so changing the measured area. Apparently also the referees of this internationally respected journal did not recognise the omission.

Limitations so far in NIRS are mostly related to the unknown and individually changing pathlength factor, the unknown vascular compartment signals are coming from and the poor and undefined spatial resolution making it hardly impossible to develop the principle into a functional imaging tool.

On the other hand NIRS displays changes in oxygenation continuous, if wanted with a temporal resolution of less than 25 ms.[26] NIRS is bedside applicable, non invasive, low cost and patient and user friendly.

References

1. Boddy SAM, Gordon AC, Thomas DFM, Browning SC. Experience with the Fowler-Stephens and microvascular procedures in the management of the intra-abdominal testes. *Br J Urol* 8: 199-202, 1991.
2. Brazy JE, Lewis DV, Mitnick MH, Jöbsis-VanderVliet FF. Noninvasive monitoring of cerebral oxygenation in preterm infants: preliminary observations. *Pediatrics* 75: 217-225,

1985.

3.   Brinkman R, Zijlstra WG, Koopmans RK. A method for continuous observation of percentage oxygen saturation in patients. *Acta Chir Neerl* 1: 333-344, 1950.

4.   Chance B, Nioka S, Kent J, McCully K, Fountain M, Greenfeld R, Holtom G. Time-resolved spectroscopy of haemoglobin and myoglobin in resting and ischemic muscle. *Anal Biochem* 174: 698-707, 1988.

5.   Colier WNJM, Meeuwissen IABE, Degens H and Oeseburg B. Determination of oxygen consumption in muscle during exercise using near infrared spectroscopy. *Acta Anaesthesiol Scand* 39 (S107): 151-155, 1995.

6.   Colier WNJM, Froeling FMJ, De Vries JDM and Oeseburg B. Measurement of the blood supply to the abdominal testis by means of near infrared spectroscopy. *Eur Urol* 27: 160-166, 1995.

7.   Colier WNJM. *Near infrared spectroscopy: toy or tool? An investigation on the clinical applicability of near infrared spectroscop.* University of Nijmegen, The Netherlands, ISBN 90-9008670-6, 1995.

8.   Colier WNJM, Binkhorst RA and Oeseburg B. Cerebral and circulatory haemodynamics before and during vasovagal syncope induced by orthostatic stress (1997). *Clin Physiol* 17: 83-94, 1997.

9.   Colier WNJM, Quaresima V, Barattelli G, Cavallari P and Ferrari M. Detailed evidence of cerebral haemoglobin oxygenation in response to motor cortical activation revealed by a continuous wave spectrophotometer with 10 Hz temporal resolution. *SPIE* 2979: 390-396, 1997.

10. Colier WNJM, Van Haaren NJHC, Van de Ven MJT, Folgering HTM and Oeseburg B. Age dependency of cerebral oxygenation assessed with near infrared spectroscopy. *J Biomed Optics* 2: 162-170, 1998.

11. De Blasi RA, Ferrari M, Natali A, Conti G, Mega A, Gasparetto A. Noninvasive measurement of forearm blood flow and oxygen consumption by near infrared spectroscopy. *J Appl Physiol* 76: 1388-1393, 1994.

12. Delpy DT, Cope M, Zee P van der, Arridge S, Wray S, Wyatt J. Estimation of optical pathlength through tissue from direct time of flight measurements. *Phys Med Biol* 33: 1433-1442, 1988.

13. Edwards AD, Wyatt JS, Richardson CE, Delpy DT, Cope M, Reynolds EOR. Cotside measurement of cerebral blood flow in ill newborn infants by near-infrared spectroscopy (NIRS). *Lancet* 2: 770-771, 1988.

14. Elwell CE, Cope M, Edwards AD, Wyatt JS, Reynolds EOR. Measurement of cerebral blood flow in adult humans using near infrared spectroscopy - methodology and possible errors. *Adv Exp Med Biol* 317: 325-245, 1992.

15. Ferrari M, Wei Q, Carraresi L, De Blasi RA, Zaccanti G. Time-resolved spectroscopy of human forearm. *J Photochem Photobiol* 16: 141-153, 1992.

16. Giannini I, Ferrari M, Carpi A, Fasella P. Rat brain monitoring by near infrared spectroscopy: an assessment of possible clinical significance. *Physiol Chem Phys* 14: 295-305, 1982.

17. Grubb BP, Gerard G, Roush K, Temesy-Armos P, Montford P, Elliott L, Hahn H, Brewster P. Cerebral vasoconstriction during head-upright tilt-induced vasovagal response. *Circulation* 84: 1157-1164, 1991.

18. Grubb BP, Orecchio E, Kurczynski TW. Head-upright tilt table testing in evaluation of recurrent, unexplained syncope. *Pediatr Neurol* 8: 423-427, 1992.

19. Harkel ten ADJ, Lieshout van JJ, Karemaker JM, Wieling W. Differences in circulatory

control in normal subjects who faint and who do not faint during orthostatic stress. *Clin Auton Res* 3: 117-123, 1993.

20. Jöbsis FF. Noninvasive , infrared monitoring of cerebral and myocardial oxygen suffiency and circulatory parameters. *Science* 198: 1264-1267, 1997.
21. Kooijman HM, Hopman MTE, Colier WNJM, Van der Vliet JA and Oeseburg B. Near infrared spectroscopy for non-invasive assessment of claudication. *J Surg Res*, 72: 1-7, 1997.
22. Liem KD, Hopman JCW, Kollée LAA , Oeseburg B. Effects of repeated indomethacin administration on cerebral oxygenation and haemodynamics in preterm infants: combined near infrared spectrophotometry and Doppler ultrasound study. *Eur J Pediatr* 153: 504-509, 1994.
23. Liem KD, Hopman JCW, Oeseburg B, de Haan AFJ, Festen C, Kollee LAA. Cerebral oxygenation and hemodynamics during induction of extracorpereal membrane oxygenation as investigated by near infrares spectroscopy. *Pediatrics* 1995.
24. Liem KD., Neonatal cerebral oxygenation and hemodynamics: A study using near infrared spectroscopy. Thesis 1996.
25. Sevick EM, Chance B, Leigh J, Nioka S, Maris M. Quantitation of time- and frequency-resolved optical spectra for the determination of tissue oxygenation. *Anal Biochem* 195: 330-351, 1991
26. Van der Sluijs MC, Colier WNJM, Houston RJF and Oeseburg B. A new and highly sensitive continuous wave near infrared spectrophotometer with multiple detectors. *SPIE*, 3194: 63-72, 1998.
27. Wyatt JS, Cope M, Delpy DT, Wray S, Reynolds EOR. Quantification of cerebral oxygenation and haemodynamics in sick newborn infants by near infrared spectroscopy. *Lancet* 2: 1063-1066, 1986.

Fos immunohistochemistry as a tool to map multisynaptic pathways activated by hypercapnia

Luc J. Teppema and J.G Veening

Introduction

During the last four decades, many studies have been devoted to the identification of central respiratory chemoreceptors. Until recently, the only brainstem area with a precise anatomical description of areas with a specific sensitivity to changes in local CO_2/H^+ concentration, is the ventrolateral medullary surface in the cat.[1] Recent studies, however, applying local injections of acidifying agents and drugs affecting synaptic transmission, indicate that central chemoreceptors may be spread more uniformly throughout the brainstem or even may be located in higher brain structures.[2,3,4,5,16] A remarkable outcome of some of these studies is that enormous ventilatory responses can be elicited by strictly localized injections of drugs and CO_2, i.e. with a radius < 350 µm.[2,3]

An alternative technique which may be useful in the localization of central chemoreceptors is Fos immunohistochemistry. In activated neurones (as in other cell types), the proto-oncogene *c-fos* is upregulated, resulting in an increased concentration of the nuclear protein-product Fos.[6,7,8] The fact that the Fos protein is located in the nucleus and has a rather long half-life,[9] permits a relatively easy additional detection of markers in the cytoplasm, so that the neurotransmitter-phenotype of Fos expressing cells can be studied. This makes Fos- immunohistochemistry very useful since the technique has the potential to increase the fundamental knowledge about the identity, location and neurochemical characteristics of neurons which are activated by hypercapnia and stimulating drugs. In recent years, the technique has been applied by various authors to map neuronal pathways activated during hypercapnia and hypoxia (for references see Teppema et al.[10]).

In a series of experiments in our lab we have compared the effects of hypoxia and hypercapnia on the expression of Fos in the brain of both awake and anesthetized rats. The rationale was that in order to identify neuronal pathways that are *specifically* involved in the response to hypercapnia, it would be useful:

(1) to compare the response to hypercapnia with that to hypoxia, and
(2) to compare the labelling pattern in awake animals with that obtained in anesthetized animals.

Methods

Experiments were performed in adult Wistar rats (200-300 g). The animals were placed in a flow-through chamber (in which carbon dioxide and oxygen tensions were measured continuously) and exposed to one of the following air mixtures: normal room air, 8% CO_2 + 20% O_2 balance N_2, or to 9% O_2 balance N_2. Prior to the exposure, one group of animals was anesthetized with a mixture of α-chloralose and urethan (70 and 700 mg/kg, respectively), while the other group was allowed to remain in the awake state.

After two hours, the animals were perfused transcardially with heparinized saline at 4 ^{0}C, followed by 4% paraformaldehyde in 0.1% phosphate buffered saline (PBS) (immediatly prior to this perfusion, the awake animals were also anesthetized with chloralose-urethan). The brains were removed, postfixed for several hours and stored overnight in 30% saccharose in 0.1 M PBS. Coronal (60 µm) sections were made with a freezing microtome. The sections were then treated immunohistochemically as described previously.[10] Analysis of the sections was performed with light microscopy.

Results

Control animals – effects of anesthesia
In several brain regions anesthesia induced increased levels of Fos. The most prominent areas were this was observed, were: the commissural and medial subnuclei of the Nucleus Tractus Solitarius (NTS) , area postrema, the A1 and C1 regions and the external lateral subnucleus of the Parabrachial Nucleus (PBel) at brainstem level, and the circumventricular organs at hypothalamic level, as well as the central Nucleus of the Amygdala (ceAMG).

Hypercapnic and hypoxic animals
Neither awake, nor anesthetized animals showed brain regions in which hypoxia *selectively* increased the expression of Fos. In many regions, however, both hypoxia and hypercapnia resulted in increased immunoreactivity. Generally, the effect of hypercapnia was larger. Brain regions selectively activated by hypercapnia both in awake and anesthetized animals were:

>   (I)   Superficial regions beneath the C1 region (i.e. cells located on the medullary surface or in very superficial layers – see figure 1);
>   (II)   Retrotrapezoid Nucleus (RTN);
>   (III)   Ventrolateral column of the mesencephalic periaqueductal gray (vlPAG);
>   (IV)   Supramammillary Nucleus, medial part (SUMm);
>   (V)   ceAMG.

Discussion

Although Fos immunohistochemistry is a useful tool to map multisynaptic pathways, it is important not to interpret its results without taking some important limitations into consideration: (1) false negative outcomes can not be excluded, since lack of Fos immunoreactivity is not necessarily associated with lack of activation. Possible different time courses of Fos mRNA and Fos protein synthesis should be kept in mind, as nicely demonstrated by Chan and Sawchenko;[11] (2) the technique is very sensitive to variations in experimental conditions due for example to non-specific stress (novelty stress, degree of handling, acclimatization to experimental room conditions, absence or presence of

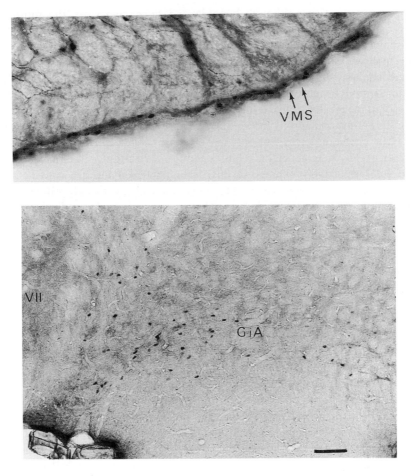

Figure 1. Expression of Fos in an awake rat exposed to 8% CO_2. Black condensed spots are nuclei stained with Fos antibody. Upper micrograph: superficial cell layers within the C1 region (i.e. within the retrofacial part of the Paragigantocellular Nucleus which is analogous to the intermediate chemosensitive area[1]). Note that the ventral medullary surface (VMS) contains several labelled cells. Lower micrograph: immunoreactive cells in the juxtafacial Paragigantocellular Nucleus and Gigantocellular Nucleus (pars alpha,GiA). VII: Facial Nucleus. Scale bar = 50 µm.

[unacquainted] congeners, etc); (3) the time pattern of Fos expression depends on the strength and duration of a given stimulus: exposure to 13 or 15% CO_2 yields significantly more labelled cells in the medulla than exposure to 8%;[10,12] (4) results on the effects of anesthesia on Fos expression should be interpreted with caution since different anesthetics have distinct effects.[13]

Apart from the above limitations, in the present study a few specific additional factors should be discussed. First, although hypoxia and hypercapnia are the most specific ventilatory stimuli available, they give also rise to a variety of hormonal and autonomic (cardiovascular) responses. However, by performing double staining to show the presence of tyrosine hydroxylase , we have shown that the labeling patterns in both catecholaminergic and non-catecholaminergic brainstem neurons after hypoxia and hypercapnia differ from those after hemodynamic challenges.[10] Second, Fos immunohistochemistry may be a valuable tool in the localization and identification of CO_2 chemoreceptors. However, Fos expression in brainstem neurons induced by hypercapnia does not prove that these cells represent CO_2 chemoreceptors, but only that they are *activated* by increased CO_2. Final identification as CO_2 chemoreceptors requires additional electrophysiological data showing that these cells, selectively expressing Fos during hypercapnia, are activated by CO_2 independently of synaptic transmission. In the hypothetical case that all cells showing Fos immunoreactivity during hypercapnia but not hypoxia were indeed specifically sensitive to CO_2, one could argue that Fos immunohistochemistry would be the most efficient means to locate and map central chemoreceptors. Our present and previous data[10] then would be the most convincing evidence for the occurrence of wide-spread chemoreceptors not only in the brainstem, but also in hypothalamic and forebrain regions. Even in the likely case that this is not true, the technique is very useful, however, since it can be combined with double staining (for example using antibodies against carbonic anhydrase, which may be a crucial enzyme in the chemosensitive mechanism).

An interesting feature of the present results is that some brainstem regions preferentially or selectively expressing Fos during hypercapnia, namely the RTN and the superficial layers beneath the C1 region (cf. the intermediate chemosensitive area[1]) are nominated as sites containing chemoreceptors.[3] Besides these areas, other nuclei such as NTS and raphe structures are also reported to contain central chemoreceptors.[2,3] The NTS shows Fos expression during both hypoxia and hypercapnia, and we have previously explained this by arguing that the location of labeled cells within the commissurual and medial subnuclei corresponds with known projection sites of carotid body afferents. This is supported by our finding that the number of immunoreactive cells was smaller in hyperoxic than in normoxic hypercapnia.[10] This does not preclude, however, the existence of CO_2 chemoreceptors in the NTS.

Another brainstem area of interest is the external lateral subnucleus of the Parabrachial Nucleus (PBel). Our previous finding in awake animals of a weak response in hypoxia but a large effect in hypercapnia[10] was confirmed by our present data. In anesthetized animals we observed a *decrease* in basal Fos expression during hypoxia, while during hypercapnia a large *increase* similar to that in awake animals was seen. Recent studies indicate that PBel may play a specific role in respiration (references see Teppema et al.[10]). It would of be of interest to investigate if the electrophysiological behavior of PBel neurons show similarities to that of RTN- and midline-neurons, and if local pharmacological manipulations (e.g. treatments with acetazolamide or glutamate antagonists) result in equally large ventilatory effects as found for these other brainstem areas.

The same is true for more rostral areas which responded specifically to CO_2, namely SUMm and ceAMG. The central Nucleus of the Amygdala contributes to excitation of the inspiratory cycle and possesses bilateral connections with respiratory brainstem areas.[14,15] The Supramammillary Nucleus, which is located somewhat more ventral and posterior to the hypothalamic sites known to be activated by hypercapnia and hypoxia,[16] responded to hypercapnia but not hypoxia. Further studies are necessary to investigate a possible role of this area in the ventilatory response to hypercapnia.

References
1. Schlaefke, ME. Central chemosensitivity: A respiratory drive. *Rev Physiol Biochem Pharmacol* 90: 171-244, 1981.
2. Bernard DG., Li A, Nattie EE. Evidence for central chemoreception in midline raphe. *J. Appl Physiol* 80: 108-115, 1996.
3. Coates EL, Li A, Nattie EE. Widespread sites of brain stem ventilatory chemoreceptors. *J Appl Physiol* 75: 5-14, 1993.
4. Dean JB, Bayliss DA, Erickson JT, Lawing WL, Millhorn DE. Depolarization and stimulation of neurons in nucleus tractus solitarii by carbon dioxide does not require chemical synaptic input. *Neuroscience* 36: 207-216, 1990.
5. Richerson GB. Response to CO_2 of neurons in the rostral ventral medulla in vitro. *J Neurophysiol*. 73: 933-944, 1995.
6. Morgan JI, Curran T. Role of ion flux in the control of *c-fos* expression. *Nature* 322: 552-555, 1986.
7. Morgan JI, Curran T. Stiumulus-transcription coupling in neurons: role of cellular immediate-early genes. *TINS* 12: 459-462, 1989.
8. Morgan JI, Curran T. Stimulus-transcription coupling in the nervous system: involvement of the inducible proto-oncogenes *fos* and *jun. Annu Rev Neurosci* 14: 421-451, 1991.
9. Morgan JI, Chen DR, Hempstead JL, Curran T. Mapping patterns of c-fos expression in the central nervous system after seizure. *Science* 237: 192-197, 1987.
10. Teppema LJ, Veening JG, Kranenburg A, Dahan A, Berkenbosch A, Olievier CN. Expression of *c-fos* in the rat brainstem after exposure to hypoxia and to normoxic and hyperoxic hypercapnia. *J Comp Neurol* 388: 169-190, 1997.
11. Chan RKW, Sawchenko PE. Spatially and temporally differentiated patterns of of c- fos expression in brainstem catecholaminergic cell groups induced by cardiovascular changes in the rat . *J Comp Neurol* 348: 433-460, 1994.
12. Sato A, Severinghaus JW, Basbaum AI. Medullary chemoreceptor neuron identification by c-fos immunohistochemistry .*J Appl Physiol* 73: 96-100, 1992.
13. Takayama K, Suzuki T, Miura M. The comparison of effects of various anesthetics on expression of Fos protein in the rat brain. *Neursci Lett* 176: 59-62, 1994.
14. Harper RM, Frysinger RC, Trelease RB Marks DJ. State-dependent alteration of respiratory cycle timing by stimulation of the central nucleus of the amygdala. *Brain Res* 306: 1-8, 1984.
15. Danielson EH, Magnuson DJ, Gray TS. The central amygdaloid nucleus innervation of the Dorsal Vagal Complex in rat: a phaseolus vulgaris leucoagglutinin lectin anterograde tracing study. *Brain Res Bull* 22: 705-715.
16. Dillon GH, Waldrop TG. In vitro responses of caudal hypothalamic neurons to hypoxia and hypercapnia. *Neuroscience* 51: 941-950, 1992

Cerebral venous PCO_2 and hypoxic ventilatory decline

Cees N. Olievier

Introduction

The measurement of the PCO_2 has always been an important issue in the study of the control of the ventilation. In gas the PCO_2 can easily be assessed with a capnograph, but in blood or cerebrospinal fluid (CSF) it is more complicated. Mostly is this performed by taking samples and analyzing them in a gas analyzer, consisting of membrane covered electrodes.

It is no point of discussion that the continuous measurement of the PCO_2 in body fluids yields more information than the sample method. Initially the Leiden Group undertook the continuous PCO_2 measurement in animal experiments with a normal-sized PCO_2 electrode and a flow-through cuvette, but the *in situ* calibration and the control of the temperature of the electrode were found to be difficult.

When a miniature PCO_2 electrode (General Electric type A 3128AB) became commercially available - around the year 1975 - we observed its performance with special interest. It showed that the electrode could be easily removed from the cuvette for (re)calibration and that the accuracy of the measurement was sufficient for research applications, when suitable corrections for drift and temperature effects were accomplished.[1,2] To our knowledge this electrode is no longer available for several years. Meant to be disposable, they function, however, still perfectly in the experiments during decades.

The electrode is used in artificial brain stem perfusion (ABP) experiments to measure continuously the PCO_2 of the 'central' and the 'peripheral' blood in cats.[3] In other experiments it measured the arterial PCO_2 in an extracorporeal circuit. The electrode assessed the cat's cerebrospinal fluid PCO_2 in ventricular-cisternal perfusion experiments.[4] Furthermore the use of the electrode for the measurement of the cerebral venous PCO_2 ($PvCO_2$) in cats is reported here.

Methods

Cats were anesthetized with a mixture of α-chloralose and urethane and part of the skull was exposed. Then a hole was drilled 15 mm rostrally from the external occipital protuberance, the superior sagittal sinus was opened and the inlet of the thermostated cuvette for the PCO_2 electrode was clamped on the hole. The cat was heparinized. Blood from the superior sagittal sinus was slowly sucked at a rate of 1 ml/min through the cuvette by means of a roller pump which returned the blood into a femoral vein. Inspiratory ventilation, in- and expiratory PCO_2 and PO_2 were measured with a Fleisch flow transducer, a capnograph and a fast-responding O_2 meter, respectively. Arterial

PCO_2 ($PaCO_2$) and PO_2 (PaO_2) were continuously measured with an extracorporeal circuit connected between a femoral artery and vein. By varying the composition of the inspired gas the blood gases were changed and the $PvCO_2$ was measured at constant $PaCO_2$ in the steady state at PaO_2 levels of about 50, 13, 6.6 and 4.0 kPa. The series of measurements was repeated with a different $PaCO_2$.

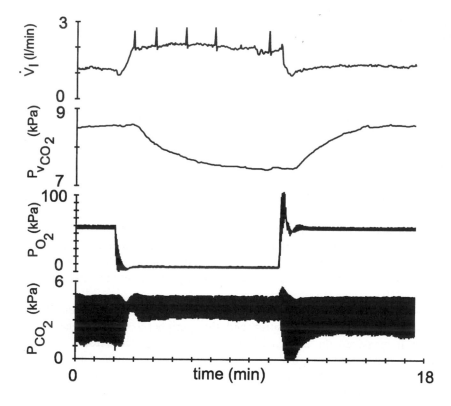

Figure 1. Example of a live tracing of $PvCO_2$ experiment. For explanation see text.

Results and Conclusions

In figure 1 a typical example of the measurement of the $PvCO_2$ is given. The lowest tracing shows the inspiratory and end-tidal PCO_2. Note that the end-tidal PCO_2 is kept as constant as possible by adjustment of the inspiratory PCO_2. The next tracing shows the inspiratory and end-tidal PO_2 with a step from hyperoxia into hypoxia and from hypoxia into hyperoxia by manipulation of the inspiratory PO_2. Then the tracing of the $PvCO_2$ is shown and it can be seen that during hypoxia the $PvCO_2$ is appreciably lowered. It must be noted that there is a time delay of the tracing due to the transport time of the venous blood from the sinus to the electrode. Moreover the time constant of the change in $PvCO_2$ is influenced by the response time of the electrode and the pump rate. The upper tracing is the ventilation on a breath-by-breath basis and the stimulation of the ventilation by the hypoxia is pronounced. The peaks in the ventilation, seen in the hypoxic period, are sighs. Note the undershoot of the ventilation at the beginning of the step into hyperoxia despite the short-lasting overshoot in end-tidal PCO_2.

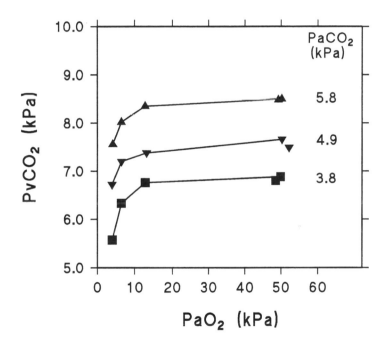

Figure 2. Example of an experiment in which the $PvCO_2$ is measured as a function of the PaO_2 at three levels of the $PaCO_2$.

Figure 2 represents the results of an experiment in which the $PvCO_2$ is measured as a function of the PaO_2 at three levels of the $PaCO_2$ (at 3.8, 4.9 and 5.8 kPa, respectively). The points in the figure are connected by straight lines. The sequence of the

End-tidal inspiratory activity and asthma

S.C.M. Luijendijk and C.P.M. van der Grinten

End-tidal inspiratory activity and hyperinflation

In quietly breathing, healthy subjects functional residual capacity (FRC) closely corresponds to relaxed lung volume. Apparently, during resting breathing end-tidal respiratory muscle activity is virtually absent, and in that condition pleural pressure (P_{PL}) and the static component of transthoracic pressure ($P_{TH\text{-}STAT}$) are equal. In a study devoted to the role of respiratory muscles in the hyperinflation of asthma, Martin et al.[1] induced different levels of hyperinflation in asymptomatic patients by doubling the dose of inhaled, aerosolized histamine and observed that at each level of hyperinflation maximum P_{PL} during expiration was generally less than predicted $P_{TH\text{-}STAT}$. They interpreted this finding to indicate persistent inspiratory muscle contraction throughout expiration. The general view at the time of this study in the late seventies was that hyperinflation in bronchial asthma was due to expiratory airflow limitation. Accordingly, Martin et al.[1] found that the increases in FRC with increasing dose of histamine were linearly correlated to the increases in pulmonary resistance. They concluded, however, that persistent activity of inspiratory muscles during expiration must have been a major determinant of the observed hyperinflation because hyperinflation occurred independently of expiratory airflow limitation.

The above conclusion is based on measurements of mechanical quantities in particular P_{PL} and $P_{TH\text{-}STAT}$, where data for $P_{TH\text{-}STAT}$ were obtained from the literature. More convincing evidence for the occurrence of persisting inspiratory activity in asthma and its role in hyperinflation was obtained from recordings of the electrical activities of inspiratory muscles. Muller et al.[2] recorded the EMG activities of the diaphragm and parasternal intercostal muscles during acute, histamine-induced hyperinflation both in healthy subjects and asymptomatic asthmatics. They found that hyperinflation was accompanied by continuation of inspiratory muscle activity during expiration, and the degree of hyperinflation correlated well with the degree of end-tidal inspiratory activity (ETIA). A similar relationship was found in asthmatics, where hyperinflation and ETIA were induced by withholding the bronchodilatory medication of the patients for 12 hours prior to the measurements[3].

Meessen et al.[4] have shown that in histamine-induced asthma in humans the larger part of the increase in FRC is due to elevated ETIA. This finding confirmed the earlier assumptions by Martin et al.[1] and Muller et al.[3]

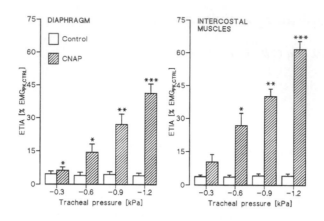

Figure 1. Effects of different levels of continuous negative airway pressure (CNAP) on end-tidal inspiratory activity (ETIA) in the diaphragm and parasternal intercostal muscles. ETIA is expressed as a percentage of mean peak EMG activity during control. Error bars indicate 1 SEM. Temperature of the cervical vagi was 37 °C. Asterisks indicate statistically significant differences compared with control (*** P<0.001; ** P<0.01; * P<0.05). (Reprinted from Meessen et al.[7]).

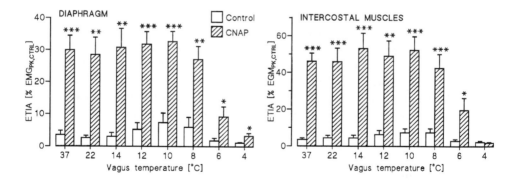

Figure 2. Effects of vagal cooling on end-tidal inspiratory activity (ETIA) in the diaphragm and parasternal intercostal muscles. ETIA was induced by a continuous negative airway pressure of -0.9 kPa. Asterisks indicate statistically significant differences compared with control at the same temperature. For further explanation see figure 1. (Reprinted from Meessen et al.[7]).

End-tidal inspiratory activity and lung receptors

Patberg[5] was the first who investigated the role of lung receptors in evoking ETIA. The experiments were performed in anaesthetized rabbits. Using positive and negative tracheal pressures (P_{TR}) relative to ambient pressure, step-by-step vagal cooling from 37 °C down to 0 °C, and vagotomy he arrived at the conclusion that ETIA is caused by a vagal reflex. He showed that ETIA is particularly evoked by application of negative P_{TR}, and that the levels of ETIA reached under that condition exceeded those reached after vagotomy. He concluded, therefore, that disinhibition of inspiratory activity by diminished activity of slowly adapting pulmonary stretch receptors (SARs) cannot be the primary cause for the observed, elevated levels of ETIA during breathing at negative P_{TR}, and he suggested that other receptors that are excited by lung deflation are involved in generating ETIA. Badier et al.[6] addressed the same issue also in rabbits. These authors applied both mechanical and chemical stimuli to provoke elevated ETIA, and procaine to block conduction in thin myelinated and non-myelinated vagal fibres. In general, the procaine block abolished the response of ETIA to the applied stimuli (inspiratory resistive loading, histamine, phenyl diguanide, and carbachol). Badier et al.,[6] therefore, concluded that this response is mediated by receptors with thin afferent fibres which include rapidly adapting pulmonary stretch receptors (RARs) and C-fibre endings.

Table 1. Stimuli used and their effects on the three different types of lung receptors. Slowly (SARs) and rapidly (RARs) adapting pulmonary stretch receptors. Temperature ranges indicate where the larger part of the conductance in the afferent fibres of the respective receptors is blocked.

Stimulus	SARs	RARs	C-fibre endings
CNAP	–	+ +	
CPAP	+ +	+	
Histamine		+ +	
Capsaine			+ +
Vagal cooling	12 - 8 °C	8 - 4 °C	< 4 °C

Meessen et al.[7,8] continued the study into the role of the different types of lung receptors in the genesis of ETIA. The experiments were performed in spontaneously breathing, anaesthetized cats. EMG electrodes were placed directly into the diaphragm and parasternal intercostal muscles (ICM). Lung receptor activity was modulated by continuous negative airway pressure (CNAP), continuous positive airway pressure (CPAP), and i.v. administrations of histamine and capsaicin. CNAP stimulates RARs and inhibits SARs. CPAP stimulates mainly SARs. Histamine stimulates RARs, and capsaicin stimulates C-fibre endings (table 1). In addition, step-by-step cooling of the cervical vagus nerves was used to selectively attenuate the central input from the

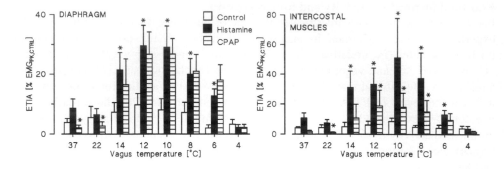

Figure 3. End-tidal inspiratory activity (ETIA) during control, after administration of histamine, and during additionally applied continuous positive airway pressure (CPAP) of 0.9 kPa at different vagus temperatures. Asterisks indicate statistically significant differences in ETIA between histamine and control values, and between CPAP(+histamine) and histamine values for that temperature. For further explanation see figure 1. (Reprinted from Meessen et al.[8]).

different types of lung receptors (table 1). Meessen et al.[7,8] mention that considerable fraction of the experimental animals did not show elevated ETIA in response to the lowest applied level of CNAP (-1.2 kPa relative to ambient pressure) or histamine (300 µg) or both. Figures 1-3, therefore, refer to the remaining responders. Figure 1 shows that ETIA, expressed as percentage of peak EMG activity of control breaths ($EMG_{PK\text{-}CTRL}$), increases with decreasing CNAP. The experimental animals were cannulated and at P_{tr} of -1.2 kPa ETIA reached, on average, a level of 50% $EMG_{PK\text{-}CTRL}$ (fig. 1).

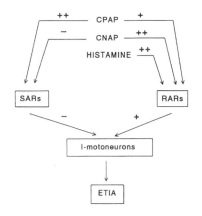

Figure 4. Schematic presentation of the effects of continuous positive airway pressure (CPAP), continuous negative airway pressure (CNAP) and histamine on slowly adapting pulmonary stretch receptor (SAR) activity and rapidly adapting pulmonary stretch receptor (RAR) activity, and of the impact of SAR and RAR activity on inspiratory motoneuron activity and end-tidal inspiratory muscle activity (ETIA). Plus and minus signs refer to stimulation and inhibition, respectively. (Reprinted from Meessen et al.[8]).

Meessen et al.[8] have further shown that histamine-induced ETIA (at normal temperature of the vagus nerves) can be attenuated by additional application of CPAP (fig. 3). Thus, CNAP and CPAP affect ETIA oppositely. In animals that responded to CNAP and histamine ETIA could no longer be evoked after vagotomy. Further, i.v. administration of capsaicin, a drug that stimulates C-fibre endings did not induce ETIA in these animals.[7,8] Latter observations imply that CNAP and histamine induce ETIA by a vagal reflex, in which C-fibre endings are not involved. Thus, the most likely origin for the observed elevation of ETIA by CNAP and histamine is excitation of inspiratory motoneuron activity through stimulation of RARs (table 1). This is supported by the results obtained by vagal cooling (figs. 2-3) which show that ETIA sharply declines between 8 and 4 °C. This is the temperature range in which the conduction of activity of RARs also sharply declines.[9] Application of CPAP decreased the level of histamine-induced ETIA at vagus temperatures of 37 °C and 22 °C (fig. 3). CPAP stimulates mainly SARs. Therefore, Meessen et al.[8] ascribed this finding to inhibition of inspiratory activity by stimulation of SARs. Accordingly, attenuation of afferent activity of SARs by cooling the vagus nerves to 14 °C or below abolished the effect of CPAP on ETIA (fig. 3). The essentials of the above discussion are shown in figure 4.

In general, hyperinflation in asthma is considered to be advantageous. An elevated lung volume enhances the delating forces of lung tissue on the airway walls thus helping to keep the airways open by opposing the broncho-constrictive forces in the airway walls. A disadvantage, however, is that the work of breathing increases by hyperinflation due to the enhanced elastic recoil of the respiratory system at elevated lung volumes. In addition, an excessive increase in FRC to levels close to total lung capacity will limit the possibilities for generating an adequate breathing pattern due to the reduced inspiratory capacity. As discussed above several authors conclude that elevated ETIA is a major determinant of hyperinflation in clinical or experimental asthma. As a consequence, during an asthmatic attack a moderate increase in ETIA may be very useful by increasing lung volume and thereby dilating the airways. On the contrary, an excessive increase in ETIA may deteriorate the clinical condition of the patient through inspiratory muscle fatigue secondary to the increased work of breathing at elevated lung volumes, and hypoventilation caused by the inability to generate an adequate breathing pattern at large lung volumes.

References
1. Martin J, Powell E, Shore S, Emrich J, Engel LA. The role of respiratory muscles in the hyperinflation of bronchial asthma. *Amer Rev Respir Dis* 121: 441-447, 1980.
2. Muller N, Bryan AC, Zamel N. Tonic inspiratory muscle activity as a cause of hyperinflation in histamine-induced asthma. *J Appl Physiol* 49: 869-874, 1980.
3. Muller N, Bryan AC, Zamel N. Tonic inspiratory muscle activity as a cause of hyperinflation in asthma. *J Appl Physiol* 50: 279-282, 1981.
4. Meessen NEL, van der Grinten CPM, Luijendijk SCM, Folgering HThM. Histamine induced bronchoconstriction and end tidal inspiratory activity in man. *Thorax* 51: 1192-1198, 1996.
5. Patberg WR. Effect of graded vagal blockade and pulmonary volume on tonic inspiratory activity in rabbits. *Pflügers Arch.* 398: 88-92, 1983.

6. Badier M, Jammes Y, Romero-Colomer P, Lemerre C. Tonic activity in inspiratory muscles and phrenic motoneurons by stimulation of vagal afferents. *J Appl Physiol* 66: 1613-1619, 1989.
7. Meessen NEL, van der Grinten CPM, Folgering HThM, Luijendijk SCM. Tonic activity in inspiratory muscles during continuous negative airway pressure. *Respir Physiol* 92: 151-166, 1993.
8. Meessen NEL, van der Grinten CPM, Folgering HThM, Luijendijk SCM. Histamine-induced end-tidal inspiratory activity and lung receptors in cats. *Eur Respir J* 8: 2094-2103, 1995.
9. Jonzon A, Pisarri TE, Roberts AM, Coleridge JCG, Coleridge HM. Attenuation of pulmonary afferent input by vagal cooling in dogs. *Respir Physiol* 72: 19-34, 1988.

Sleep disordered breathing in patients with chronic obstructive pulmonary disease

H. Folgering, P. Vos, Y. Heijdra, M. Wagenaar and C. v. Herwaarden

Introduction

Nocturnal hypoxia often occurs in patients with chronic obstructive pulmonary disease (COPD). In a group of 60 patients with an FEV_1 below 65% of the reference value, we found episodes of desaturation in 47 patients (78%).[1] Control of breathing during sleep depends highly on the sleep-stage. In non-REM sleep (nREM; no rapid eye movements) the 'metabolic' control of breathing is intact: ventilation (V_I) is regulated to a level where the need of oxygen uptake and the elemination of carbon dioxide is met. There is an absence of the 'wakefullness drive', which leads to some hypoventilation and lowered responsiveness to hypoxia, and especially to hypercapnia (fig. 1). The arterial PCO_2 is usually increased by 0.5 to 1.0 kPa, as compared to the awake state.[2] Nevertheless, the major ventilatory drive in slow wave sleep is the CO_2 drive.

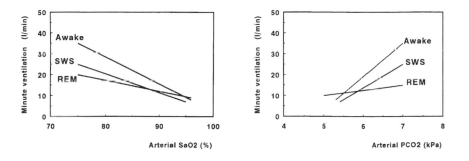

Figure 1. Ventilatory responses to hypercapnia (right) and to hypoxia (left) during wakefulness, Slow Wave Sleep (SWS) and REM sleep.

In stage 1 nREM, which lasts only a for a few minutes, there are some instabilities in the control of breathing, giving rise to a Cheyne Stokes type of breathing. Some severe COPD-patients show this type of breathing even when awake. During nREM stages 2, 3 and 4, breathing becomes very regular, more regular than in the awake state. During SWS (nREM stages 3 and 4), the tone of respiratory muscles is decreased; consequently the neuro-mechanical coupling is lowered, leading to further hypoventilation. There is also a loss of tone of the upper pharyngeal muscles that results in an increased upper airway resistance. This also may alter the ventilatory responses to hypoxia and hypercapnia. The loss of tone of upper pharyngeal muscles during sleep may lead to substantial problems in obese COPD-patients; it may induce episodes of sleep apnea. The combined occurrence of any pulmonary disease (COPD, Cystic Fibrosis, Ideopathic Pulmonary fibrosis) and sleep apnea syndrome leads to further nocturnal desaturations, and is called: "overlap syndrome".[3]

Diagnosis

During phasic REM-sleep, breathing becomes irregular, often with erratic patterns, and is probably somewhat more influenced by 'behavioural mechanisms' which occur during dreaming in REM-sleep. Due to the 'gamma-paralysis' there is no activity in the intercostal muscles. Consequently, the diaphragm is virtually the only respiratory muscle that is active during REM sleep. This leads to paradoxical breathing and further hypoventilation. During tonic REM, the breathing pattern is fairly regular, and predominantly diaphragmatic.

In COPD, the diaphragm is chronically flattened, and consequently on a disadvantageous position on its length-tension curve. The insertional force of the diaphragm that raises the lower costal margins in normals, is directed more in the transverse direction, making the diaphragmatic contractions more of an expiratory nature, and less efficient. Furthermore, respiratory muscles are frequently weakened in COPD patients, related to the level of hyperinflation.[4] In the supine position, the strengh

Table 1

Sleep Stage	NREM 1,2	NREM 3,4	REM tonic	REM phasic
Regulation	metabolic	metabolic	behavioural	metabolic
Breathing pattern	periodic regular	regular	(ir)regular	irregular
Ventilatory Responses to O_2 and CO_2	low	low	lower	lowest (or absent)
Upper airway resistance	normal	higher	higher	highest
Ribcage movement	normal	normal (increased)	low	absent
Abdominal movement	normal (decreased)	decreased	absent	absent or paradoxical
Minute ventilation	somewhat low	low	lowest	variable
Pa_{CO_2}	somewhat high	higher	highest	variable
Pa_{O_2}	somewhat low	lower	lowest	variable

of the inspiratory muscles decreases even further.[5] Finally, the FRC will be lower in the supine position, thus reducing the oxygen store in the lungs, and increasing ventilation-perfusion mismatches. All this will contribute to possible hypoxemia especially during REM sleep in COPD patients (table 1).

Many patients suffering from COPD, also use diuretics for a concomittant heart failure or peripheral edema of other origin. Especially loop diuretics generate a metabolic alkalosis, and thus diminish one of the important ventilatory drives. This will make the nocturnal hypoventilation more severe. The same holds for sedatives; the central ventilatory depression that these drugs induce, will cause nocturnal hypoxia in COPD-patients to deepen.

The consequences of nocturnal hypoxemia in patients with COPD is not really clear. Some animal experiments suggest that 2/24 hrs of desaturation to PaO_2-levels of approximately 7.5 kPa suffices for developement of pulmonary hypertension.[6]. This seems to be partially supported by the findings of Fletcher,[7] suggesting that nocturnal desaturations might shorten life expectancy in patients with COPD. In the acute situation during nocturnal desaturations to 94-77%, there are indeed transient rises in pulmonary artery pressure.[8] On the other hand, Connaughton and coworkers[9] did not find any justification in monitoring nocturnal oxygen saturation in patients with COPD, and giving some of them oxygen during the night. A recent study by Chaouat et al.[10] showed that COPD-patients with hypoxemia only during sleep, do not have pulmonary hypertension.

Nocturnal hypoxemia, ventilatory effort, and especially hypercapnia disturbs the normal sleep architecture:[11,12] the distribution of the various phases of sleep, resulting in reduced cognitive functioning (Bourdon-Vos pattern-recognition test) and neuropsychological functioning, and even psychomotor functioning (finger tapping).[13,14] The movement arousal index in COPD-patients was normal.[15]

Diagnosis

Daytime blood gas values are related to nocturnal hypoxaemia in groups of patients.[16] Especially the blue and bloating type of COPD-patients seem to desaturate during the night.[3] This relationship between daytime PaO_2 holds for groups of patients (r = 0.56,[17] r = 0.81,[18]). However, for the individual case, the predictive value of a daytime bloodgas analysis hardly is relevant at these levels of correlation. Using daytime bloodgas values for predicting nocturnal saturation would miss this phenomenon in 20% of the COPD patients, and 22% would be falsely diagnosed as nocturnal desaturators. Measuring also the ventilatory respones to CO_2 in these patients improves the negative predictive value for nocturnal hypoxaemia to 91%, the positive predictive value remains low at 50%.[17]

Exercise also causes desaturations in severe COPD-patients. The hypoxia of exercise was a good predictor of nocturnal desaturations (r = 0.81), but not as good as daytime resting PaO_2.[18]

One of the causes of nocturnal saturations is the starting position of the patient's PaO_2 on the shoulder of the oxygen desaturation curve, makes that a relatively modest decrease in PaO_2 immediately shows in a fall in saturation, whereas the same fall in PaO_2

from a higher starting point on the horizontal part of the dissociation curve will not be accompanied by a desaturation.The saturation pattern of the COPD-patient is very characteristic, and differs substantially from e.g. the pattern in obstructive sleep apnea. The desaturating COPD-patient shows three to four episodes of desaturation, lasting 30-45 minutes, and are approximately 1.5 hrs apart (fig. 2). This is in contrast to the patients with Obstructive Sleep apnea, who show a saw-tooth like sturation pattern, returning to (near) normal saturations between the obstructions.

The basic problem of these nocturnal desaturations in COPD patients is hypoventilation during REM sleep. Thus the primary deviating parameter is arterial P_{CO_2}. This can be measured by sampling from an indwelling arterial catheter. Such an invasive measurement can be avoided by measuring end-tidal P_{CO_2}. Its absolute value is not equivalent to the arterial values in COPD, however changes in $P_{ET}CO_2$ do reflect changes in Pa_{CO_2}. Measuring $P_{ET}CO_2$ in COPD patients will show hypoventilation, also in patients who do not desaturate.[19]

Measuring trancutaneous P_{CO_2} is another possibility for detecting hypoventilations. P_{CO_2} electrodes are notoriously slow (responsetime 2-3 min, risetime 1.5 min), and should be heated to approximately 42 °C. Therefore, the electrodes cannot be left on the same site of skin for more than 4 hours.

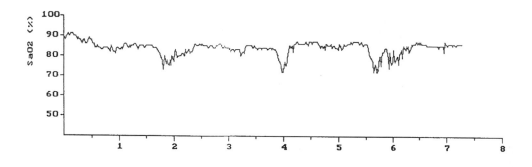

Figure 2. Nocturnal saturation pattern in a COPD patient. Horizontal axis: hours sleep time. Vertical axis: saturation measured by pulse oximetry.

Airflow usually is measured with thermistors in front of the nose and mouth. The changes in temperatures of the passing air cannot exceed the range between 37 °C and ambient temperature. Thus this is only a qualitative measurement of V_I: presence or absence of airflow. Hypoventilation cannot be diagnosed with this device. Breathing efforts can be measured by respiratory inductive plethysmography, or by EMG-activity of the respiratory muscles. Sleep stages should be assessed by EEG, and/or EOG. Video monitoring will suffice to show movement-arousals and parasomnia's such as periodic leg movements.

Therapy

Treatment can be performed in a number of ways, ranging from nocturnal oxygen suppletion, to non-invasive ventilation, pharmacologic treatment with respiratory stimulants, and to inspiratory muscle training. As decribed above, there is still some controversy on the clinical need to correct isolated nocturnal hypoxaemia in COPD patients. More and more evidence is accumulating that these nocturnal isolated incidences of hypoxaemia do not lead to devolopement of pulmonary hypertension. The latter is associated with a low survival rate. Chaouat et al.[10] performed a multi-center study on 94 COPD-patients who were normoxic at daytime: 66 nocturnal desaturators and 28 non-desaturators. Both groups showed the same pulmonary artery pressures. Nocturnal desaturation was associated with higher daytime $PaCO_2$ (6.0 *vs.* 5.3; P <0.001) but surprisingly not with daytime PaO_2 (8.4 *vs.* 8.4 kPa; NS). These authors did not firmly conclude that supplying oxygen during the night will do nothing to prevent the developement of pulmonary hypertension. A longitudinal study is on its way.

In the perspective of these uncertainties, one might still rightfully consider to improve nocturnal oxygenation in patients with COPD with daytime and nocturnal desaturations. According to the standards for COPD of the American Thoracic Society (ATS) and the European Respiratory Society (ERS), there still remains the indication for providing supplemental oxygen for more than 15 hours per day, if the stable daytime PaO_2 is lower than 7.3 kPa or SaO_2 < 88%.[20,21]

Administering supplemental oxygen during sleep is very effective in improving nocturnal saturation. It increased by 7.4%, as compared to compressed air, in Vos' study.[29] However, also $PaCO_2$ increased by 0.6 kPa, due to a diminished peripheral chemoreceptor stimulation. The same improvements in nocturnal saturation were found by Damato et al.[30], in a similar cross over study where oxygen or compressed air was given to COPD patients during the night.

The role of chronic (nocturnal) non-invasive ventilation in very severe COPD patients still remains to be established.[21,22] The aim of such treatment would be either resting the overexerted respiratory muscles, or 'resetting' the control of breathing by artificially lowering arterial PCO_2 for a certain period. In periods of exacerbations, oxygen therapy or transient non-invasive ventilation can be required, and it will improve the prognosis of the patient. In a randomised study, 60 COPD-patients with an exacerbation were assigned to conventional treatment with or without nasal ventilation. In the ventilated group 3/30 did not survive, versus 9/30 in the conventionally treated group.[22]

Pharmacological stimulation of V_I can be performed by progesterone, acetazolamide, Doxapram, Almitrine, theophylline or protryptilline. Such a medication, can only be usefull if the ventilatory pump is capable of generating a higher V_I, and thus capable of eleminating more CO_2. This can be tested by voluntary hyperventilation and monitoring the end-tidal PCO_2. If a patient can 'blow off' extra CO_2, and thus can lower $P_{ET}CO_2$, it is reasonable to assume that the ventilatory muscles are able to effectuate an increased ventilatory drive, for at least a short period. Doxapram can only be given intravenously, and therefore can only be used in acute clinical situations.[23] Progesterone effects on V_I are mediated by the hypothalamus. The stimulating effect of this drug is eliminated after midcollicular decerebration in cats.[24] Medroxyprogesterone acetate stimulates V_I in patients with CO_2-retention, and increases the ventilatory responses.[25] Another synthetic progesterone derivative, chlormadinone acteate, lowers $PaCO_2$ by 0.7 kPa, and increased mean nocturnal saturation by 2.1% in a group of 18 COPD patients. The ventilatory response to CO_2 increases from 2.3 to 3.3 $l.min^{-1}.kPa^{-1}$. There is no effect on the ventilatory response to hypoxia.[29]

The inhibitor of carbonic anhydrase, acetazolamide, induces a metabolic acidosis, and thus stimulates V_I. In anesthetised cats, this is mediated by a leftward shift of the ventilatory response curve to CO_2. Both central and peripheral chemoreflex loops seem to be less sensitive in such a preparation. Modelling ventilatory control, and using a mass balance for CO_2 in the brain compartment, it seems likely that acetazolamide also has its effects on cerebral blood flow.[26] In awake human COPD patients, the situation seems to be different from anesthetised cats: the slope of the ventilatory reponse curves to CO_2 increased from 0.2 to 1.0 $l.min^{-1}.kPa^{-1}$, and the slope of the ventilatory response to hypoxia increased from 0.05 to 0.12 $l.min^{-1}.(\%\ desaturation)^{-1}$ in a group of COPD patients. Nocturnal oxygen saturation improved by 4.3%. Desaturation time decreased by 30.0 minutes. Surprising, but difficult to explain, was the improvement in total sleep time by 2.2 hours, after giving acetazolamide to these patients.[29]

Theophylline has a central stimulating effect on V_I; it probably improves muscle contractility, and causes a bronchodilation. Mulloy[27] administered this drug to 10 COPD patients. The mean nocturnal oxygen saturation improved by 2%, and the mean $PtcCO_2$ was lowered by 0.5 kPa. Theophylline was tested versus salbutamol in a randomised double blind cross over study in 19 COPD patients, on its effects on nocturnal respiratory function and sleep quality. The latter was not different between both drugs. The sleep time spent in saturation levels below 90% was 72 minutes during salbutamol, and 51 minutes during theophylline ($P = 0.03$).[28]

Inspiratory muscle training can be used for strengthening the ventilatory muscles. If appropriate training methods are used, such as targetted training or threshold loading, the maximal transdiaphragmatic pressure can improve from 6.6 to 10.0 kPa. In the same time, mean nocturnal saturation improved from 88.8% to 90.7%. The duration of the desaturation time decreased from 18.6% to 5.4% of total sleep time.[31]

Conclusion

Nocturnal breathing in more severe COPD patients is often insufficient to maintain normal blood gas values. This is due to normal mechanisms that are also active in healthy subjects. Additional problems in COPD-patients are: ventilatory muscle dysfunction, ventilation-perfusion mismatching, and defective ventilatory control. In a subgroup of patients, desaturations occur only during the night.It is still under debate whether these patients should be treated. If one decides to treat nocturnal hypoxaemia in COPD-patients, one can use respiratory stimulants, supplemental oxygen, or inspiratory muscle training. The place of chronic non invasive ventilation in very severe patients, remains to be established. Most probably, it is usefull in acute exacerbations in severe COPD.

References
1. Vos PJE, Folgering H, Herwaarden CLA van. Prevalence of oxygen desaturations and associated breathing disorders during sleep in patients with chronic obstructive pulmonary disease. In: Sleep and health risk. J.Peter, T.Penzel, T.Podzus, P.v.Wichert eds. Springer Verlag Berlin 1991, pp 246-250
2. Stradling JR. Handbook of sleep related breathing disorders. Oxford university press 1993
3. Flenley DC. Sleep in chronic obstructive lung disease. *Clin Chest Med.* 1985 ; 6: 651-661
4. Rochester DF, Braun NMT. Determinants of maximal inspiratory pressure in chronic obstructive pulmonary disease. *Am Rev Respir Dis* 1985; 132: 42-72
5. Heijdra YF, Dekhuijzen PNR, Herwaarden CLA van, Folgering H. Effects of body position hyperinflation, and blood gas tensions on maximal respiratory pressures in patients with chronic obstructive pulmonary disease. *Thorax* 1994; 49: 453-458
6. Nattie EE, Doble EA. Threshold of hypoxia induced right ventricular hypertrophy in the rat. *Respir Physiol* 1984; 56: 253-259
7. Fletcher EC, Donner CF, Midgren B, Zielinski J, Levi-Valensi P, Braghiroli A, Rida Z, Miller CC. Survival in COPD patients with a daytime PaO_2 > 60 mmHg, and without nocturnal oxyhemoglobin desaturation. *Chest* 1992; 101: 649-655
8. Boysen PG, Block JA, Wynne JW, Hunt LA, Flick MR. Nocturnal pulmonary hypertension in patients with chronic obstructive pulmonary disease. *Chest* 1979; 75: 535-542
9. Connaughton JJ, Caterall JR, Elton RA, Stradling JR, Douglas NJ. Do sleep studies contribute to the management of patients with severe obstructive pulmonary disease? *Am Rev Respir Dis* 1988; 138: 341-344
10. Chaouat A, Weitzenblum E, Kessler R, Charpentier C, Ehrhart M, Levi-Valensi P, Zielinski J, Delaunois L, Cornudella R, Moutinho dos Santos J. Sleep related desaturation and daytime pulmonary haemodynamics in COPD-patients with mild hypoxaemia. *Eur Respir J* 1997; 10:1730-1735
11. Brezinova V, Catterall JR, Douglas NJ, Calverley PMA, Flenley DC. Night sleep of patients with ventilatory failure and age-matched controls: numbers and duration of EEG episodes of intervening wakefullness and drowsiness. *Sleep* 1982; 52: 123-130
12. Gleeson K, Zwillich CW, White DP. The influence of increasing ventilatory effort on arousal from sleep. *Am Rev Respir Dis* 1190; 142: 295-300
13. Vos PJE, Folgering HTM, Herwaarden CLA van. Visual attention in patients with chronic obstructive pulmonary disease. *Biol Psychol* 1995; 41: 295-305
14. Roehrs T, Merrion M, Petrosi B, Stepanski E, Zorick F, Roth T. Neuropsychological function in obstructive sleep apnea syndrome (OSAS) compared to chronic obstructive pulmonary disease (COPD). *Sleep* 1995; 18: 382-388
15. Collard P, Dury M, Delguste P, Aubert G, Rodenstein DO. Movement arousals in sleep related disordered breathing in adults. *Am J Respir Crit Care Med* 1996; 154: 454-459
16. Douglas NJ, Flenley DC. Breathing during sleep in patients with chronic obstructive lung disease. *Am Rev Respir Dis.* 1990; 141: 1055-1070
17. Vos PJE, Folgering H, Herwaarden CLA van. Predictors for nocturnal hypoxaemia (mean SaO_2 < 90%) in normoxic and mildly hypoxic patients with COPD. *Eur Respir J* 1995; 8: 74-77
18. Mulloy E, McNicholas W. Ventilation and gas exchange during sleep and exercise in severe COPD. *Chest* 1996; 109: 387-394
19. Vos PJE, Herwaarden CLA van, Folgering H. Nocturnal end-tidal PCO_2 recordings in patients

with chronic obstructive pulmonary disease or sleep apnea syndrome. *Physiol Meas* 1993; 14: 433-439

20. American Thoracic Society. Standards for the diagnosis and care of patients with chronic obstructive pulmnoary disease and asthma. *Am J Respir Crit Care Med* 1995; 152 (suppl 5): 588-593

21. Siafakas NM, Vermeire P, Pride NB, Paoletti P, Gibson J et al. Optimal assessment and management of chronic obstructive pulmonary disease (COPD). ERS consensus statement. *Eur Respir J* 1995; 8: 1398-1420

22. Bott J, Carroll M, Conway J, Moxham J. Randomised controlled trial of nasal ventilation in acute repsiratory failure due to chronic obstructive airways disease. *Lancet* 1993; 341: 1555-1557

23. Riordan JF, Sillett RW, McNicoll MW. A controlled trial of Doxapram in acute respiratory failure. Br J Dis Chest 1975; 69: 57-62

24. Bayliss DA, Milhorn DE. Central neural mechanisms of progesterone action:application to the respiratory system. *J Appl Physiol* 1995; 27: 551-557

25. Skatrud JB, Dempsey JA. Relative effectiveness of acetazolamide versus medroxyprogesterone in correction of chronic carbon dioxide retention. *Am Rev Respir Dis* 1983; 127: 405-412

26. Wagenaar M, Teppema L, Berkenbosch A, Olievier K, Folgering H. The effect of low dose acetazolamide on the ventilatory CO_2-response curve in the anaesthetized cat. *J Physiol (Lond)* 1996; 495: 227-237

27. Mulloy E, McNicholas W. Theophylline improves gas exchange during rest, exercise and sleep in severe chronic pulmonary disease. *Am Rev Respir Dis* 1993; 148: 1030-1036

28. Man GCW, Chapman KR, Habib Ali S, Darke AC. Sleep quality and nocturnal respiratory function with once daily theophylline and inhaled salbutamol in patients with COPD. *Chest* 1996; 110: 648-653

29. Vos PJE, Herwaarden CLA van, Boo Th de, Lemmens W, Folgering H. Effects of acetazolamide, chlormadinone acetate, and oxygen on awake and asleep gas exchange in COPD-patients. *Eur Respir J* 1994; 7: 850-855

30. Damato S, Frigo V, Dell'Oca M, Negretto GG, Tarsia P. Utility of monitoring breathing during night hours in COPD patients undergoing long term oxygen therapy. *Monaldi Arch Chest Dis* 1997; 52: 106-111

31. Heydra Y, Dekhuijzen P, Herwaarden CLA van, Folgering H. Target flow inspiratory muscle training improves nocturnal saturation in patients with COPD. *Am J Respir Crit Care Med* 1996; 153: 260-265

Sleep apnea syndrome as extreme condition of the respiratory control system

Joost G. van den Aardweg, Reindert P. van Steenwijk and John M. Karemaker

Introduction

Control of respiration is hampered by the mechanics of the respiratory system: only once per breath can the respiratory control system adapt to changing input signals (chemoreception) or changing demands like increased muscular work. This implies an inevitable instability of pulmonary capillary P_{CO_2} and P_{O_2}, leading to cyclic changes in synchrony with inspiratory and expiratory movements. In addition, chemoreflexes act only after a delay to changes in pulmonary gas tensions due to the circulatory delay from the lungs to the areas of chemoreception. Thus, in spite of the availability of continuous stimuli to chemoreceptors, both the delays of afferent information and the nature of the effector organ can lead to (slower) oscillations in the respiratory control system, with periods of several or more breaths.

The respiratory control system does not only have fast chemoreflex feedback through peripheral chemoreceptors but also a slower feedback through sensory neurons in the medulla oblongata. As a result both fast and slow oscillations in respiratory effort might originate. How the time delays and amplitudes of effects characterize these two control systems has beautifully been described in the studies of Berkenbosch et al.[1-4] On the basis of these data of the dynamics of chemoreflexes it can be expected that mild respiratory oscillations can occur in healthy subjects. More pronounced oscillations of the same systems, however, may be implicated in pathologic conditions, such as the sleep apnea syndrome.

Respiratory oscillations in sleep apnea syndrome

During sleep the respiratory system seems to have a larger tendency to oscillatory patterns, which occurs in an extreme form in the sleep apnea syndrome (SAS).[5] Patients with SAS often stop breathing during sleep, mostly for more than 15 s, which can be due to either absent respiratory effort or obstruction of the higher airways (central or obstructive type). Isolated sleep apneas seldom occur. In almost every patient they are part of an oscillatory breathing pattern with apneas which repeat every 40 to 60 s. This is mostly accompanied by moderate to severe oscillations of arterial P_{CO_2} and P_{O_2} with the same periodicity. There may therefore exist a same pathogenetic mechanism in sleep apnea as in other pronounced oscillatory breathing patterns, like Cheyne-Stokes respiration.[6] Figure 1 shows an example of repetitive apneas during sleep in a patient with the obstructive type of the syndrome. The apneas lead to severe periodic desaturations (down to 70 %) as demonstrated by the pulse oximeter signal. The figure also shows the effects of the apneic breathing pattern on blood

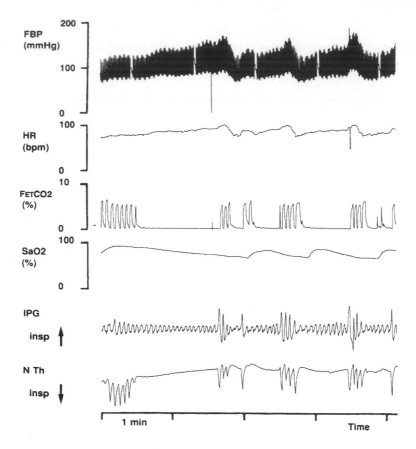

Figure 1. Recurrent apneas in a patient with obstructive sleep apnea syndrome. FBP, finger blood pressure measured by Finapres™. Short interruptions in the signal are due to automatic set-point checks of the device (Physiocal™). HR, heart rate obtained from the ECG by a cardiotachometer. FETCO$_2$, end-tidal CO$_2$ fraction of air sampled at the nose. SaO$_2$, arterial oxygen saturation as measured by pulse oximetry. IPG, impedance pneumogram, derived from thoracic ECG electrodes. Nth, nose thermistor signal. Note the long and recurrent cessations in nasal airflow as evidenced by the nose thermistor and capnograph signal, with severe desaturations and periodic changes in blood pressure and heart rate.

pressure (BP) and heart rate (HR). Both increase gradually during each apnea and decrease shortly thereafter. We found in a group of 12 SAS-patients a marked oscillation in BP and HR in association with the apneic breathing pattern.[7] Such hemodynamic instability in SAS may be involved in the genesis of the long-term cardiovascular complications of the syndrome. In an echocardiographic study of SAS patients, sleep apnea appeared to be an independent risk factor for increased left ventricular mass (independent of daytime BP

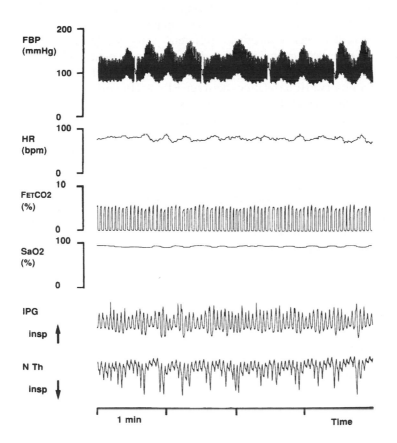

Figure 2. Moderate periodic breathing during sleep in a patient with sleep apnea syndrome. Legends as in figure 1.

level).[8] One may therefore speculate that such periodic increases in BP during or shortly after apneas are responsible for the development of left-ventricular hypertrophy in some patients. In addition, a strong epidemiological relation between SAS and daytime hypertension has been found.[9] Recent experiments in dogs have shown that imposed apneas during sleep can induce daytime hypertension, which resolves after several nights of normal sleep.[10] This interesting finding implies that an apneic breathing pattern during sleep may be the cause of a considerable number of cases of "essential" hypertension where the sleep apnea syndrome is also present. This shows that the study of respiratory oscillations may have important implications for several questions in circulatory pathophysiology. The mechanism by which sleep apneas may lead to daytime hypertension is, however, not known. More insight has been obtained in the mechanisms of acute cardiovascular effects of apneas. In healthy subjects, BP elevations during repetitive apneas appeared to be eliminated by pharmacological ganglionic blockade, implying a neural (sympathetic) mechanism.[11] We think that such sympathetic (efferent) activity may be originated in periodic stimulation of peripheral chemoreceptors during repetitive apneas, since we could eliminate apneic BP elevations in healthy subjects by inhalation of 100% O_2.[12] This hypothesis fits with the observed time relations between BP and HR during repetitive apneas in SAS patients.[7] We could simulate these time relations by a mathematical model based on the efferent vagal and sympathetic effects of the peripheral chemoreflex on the circulation. These effects mainly consist of vagal modulation of HR and sympathetic modulation of peripheral vascular resistance. In contrast, the time relations between BP and HR during apneas could not be explained by a model that describes the baroreflex response of changes in BP on vagal and sympathetic efferents. We therefore hypothesize that periodically increased chemoreflex activity due to periodic hypoxia somehow represses the baroreflex from the efferent pathways of the autonomic nervous system. This implies that chemoreflexes may not only be involved in the genesis of periodic breathing patterns, but in the genesis of circulatory sequelae as well.

Respiratory oscillations in healthy subjects

Apart from repetitive apneas, a breathing pattern of moderate waxing and waning of respiratory effort is often observed in SAS patients. This is shown in figure 2, a recording made in a sleeping patient with obstructive SAS, who did not have apneas at that time. It shows a periodic change in the amplitude of the nose thermistor and impedance pneumography signal, associated with a slight fluctuation of the pulse oximeter signal. Note that BP and HR also change with the same periodicity. In this respect, there are similarities with the periodic apneic breathing pattern, although the changes are less pronounced. We observed such patterns in many SAS patients, mostly during sleep, yet it is not clear to whether this should be considered as pathological. Some authors have found an increased tendency to (moderate) periodic breathing patterns in SAS, even during wakefulness.[13] On the basis of the abovementioned instability of the chemoreflex loops, we expect that a moderate form of periodic breathing can occur in many healthy humans. In a group of healthy students, we found indeed moderate oscillatory changes in ventilation and end-tidal CO_2 when they were quietly breathing during 30 min.[9] The repetition rate of these oscillations was in the same range as that of periodic apneas in SAS. This suggests that the same system that is responsible for the respiratory instability in SAS is also at work, albeit in a moderate manner, in healthy subjects. That normal subjects have the potential to develop pronounced periodic breathing patterns as well, is known for years from high altitude physiology and has clearly been demonstrated by experiments where periodic, even apneic, breathing patterns have been induced by hypoxia.[14]

In conclusion, our studies in sleep apnea patients and healthy subjects have demonstrated the importance of understanding the properties of the feedback systems that regulate essential homeostatic mechanisms. Phenomena like sleep apnea, Cheyne-Stokes breathing, and moderate ventilatory periodicities in healthy subjects at rest may all be governed by the same feedback properties of the respiratory control system. Only by the work of basic researchers in integrative physiology can such insight be obtained. This article is intended to honour one of these physiologists, a master in an underestimated art.

References
1. Berkenbosch A, De Goede J, Ward DS, Olievier CN, Van Hartevelt J. Dynamic response of peripheral chemoreflex loop to changes in end-tidal CO_2. *J Appl Physiol* 64: 1779 - 1785, 1988.
2. Berkenbosch A, Ward DS, Olievier CN, De Goede J, Van Hartevelt J. Dynamics of ventilatory response to step changes of PCO_2 of blood perfusing the brain stem. *J Appl Physiol* 66: 2168 - 2173, 1989.
3. Berkenbosch A, De Goede J, Ward DS, Olievier CN, Van Hartevelt J. Dynamic response of the peripheral chemoreflex loop to changes in end-tidal O_2. *J Appl Physiol* 71: 1123- 1128, 1991.
4. Berkenbosch A, Dahan A, De Goede J, Olievier ICW. The ventilatory response to CO_2 of the peripheral and central chemoreflex loop before and after sustained hypoxia in man. *J Physiol (Lond)* 456: 71 - 83, 1992.
5. Van den Aardweg JG, Karemaker JM. Respiratory variability and associated cardiovascular changes in adults at rest. *Clin Physiol Oxf* 11: 95 - 118, 1991.
6. Longobardo GS, Gothe B, Goldman MD, Cherniack NS. Sleep apnea considered as a control system instability. *Respir Physiol* 50: 311 - 333, 1982.
7. Van den Aardweg JG, Van Steenwijk RP, Karemaker JM. A chemoreflex model of relation between blood pressure and heart rate in sleep apnea syndrome. *Am J Physiol* 268 (*Heart Circ Physiol* 37): H2145 - H2156, 1995.
8. Hedner J, Ejnell H, Caidahl K. Left ventricular hypertrophy independent of hypertension in patients with obstructive sleep apnea. *J Hypertens* 8: 941 - 946, 1990.
9. Van den Aardweg JG. Cardiovascular effects of cyclic changes in breathing pattern: a study in sleep apnea patients and healthy subjects. Thesis. University of Amsterdam, 1992.
10. Brooks D, Horner RL, Kozar LF, Render-Teixeira CL, Phillipson EA. Obstructive sleep apnea as a cause of systemic hypertension: evidence from a canine model. *J Clin Invest* 99: 106 - 109, 1997.
11. Katragadda S, Xie A, Puleo D, Skatrud JB, Morgan BJ. Neural mechanism of the pressor response to obstructive and nonobstructive apnea. *J Appl Physiol* 83: 2048 - 2054, 1997.
12. Van den Aardweg JG, Karemaker JM. Repetitive apneas induce periodic hypertension in normal subjects through hypoxia. *J Appl Physiol* 72: 821 - 827, 1992.
13. Pack AI, Silage DA, Millman RP, Knight H, Shore ET, Chung DC. Spectral analysis of ventilation in elderly subjects during sleep. *J Appl Physiol* 64: 1257- 1267, 1988.
14. Chadha TS, Birch S, Sackner MA. Periodic breathing triggered by hypoxia in normal awake adults. *Chest* 88: 16 - 23, 1985.

Children who forget to breathe: the physiological enigma of the congenital central hypoventilation syndrome

David Gozal

Definition

Congenital central hypoventilation syndrome (CCHS; Ondine's Curse) is traditionally defined as the failure of automatic control of breathing.[1-10] The term "Ondine's curse" was initially coined in 1962 by Severinghaus and Mitchell to describe a syndrome manifested in 3 adult patients after high cervical/ brainstem surgery.[11] When awake and summoned to breathe, these patients would do so, but otherwise would require mechanical ventilation for severe central apnea.[11]

In CCHS, ventilation ($\dot{V}_I$) is most severely affected during quiet sleep, a state during which automatic neural control is predominant.[5] Ventilatory patterns are also abnormal during active sleep and even during wakefulness, although to a milder degree.[1,3,5,6,12-14] Severity of respiratory dysfunction may range from relatively mild hypoventilation during quiet sleep with fairly good alveolar ventilation during wakefulness, to complete apnea during sleep with severe hypoventilation during wakefulness. Other symptoms indicative of brainstem dysfunction may be present, but are not essential to make the diagnosis of CCHS.

The proposed diagnostic criteria for CCHS include all of the following:[10]

1. Persistent evidence of sleep hypoventilation ($P_aCO_2 > 60$ mmHg).
2. The onset of symptoms occurred during the first year of life.
3. Absence of primary pulmonary disease or neuromuscular dysfunction, which could explain the hypoventilation.
4. No evidence of cardiac disease.

Pathophysiology

The exact pathophysiology of CCHS remains unknown, and has been the subject of intense speculation and research. Since an extensive review of CCHS is beyond the scope of this paper, I will briefly summarize the more recent developments and current understanding on this medically challenging syndrome.

Genetic Hypothesis

CCHS could be the result of an interaction between the environment and genetics. The rationale for CCHS containing a genetic component is its early manifestation in the newborn period, its occurrence in families, and its association with Hirschsprung's disease (HSCR).[13-21] In fact, greater than 20% of reported cases of CCHS are accompanied by HSCR,[17] such that the association of these two relatively rare clinical entities suggests a possible common

65

pathogenetic basis. Since a mutation in the RET-protooncogene is associated with HSCR,[22,23] and since RET may play a critical role in the development of the neural crest and parasympathetic system in both HSCR[24] and CCHS,[25-28] a genetic screening of RET mutations was performed by several research groups with overall disappointing results.[29-31] Similarly, mutations in the endothelin gene were described in a patient with CCHS,[32] although the significance of such finding remains yet to be established. It should be emphasized that the putative genetic etiology of CCHS is at least partially undermined by the fact that family members of CCHS do not display any evidence of respiratory control dysfunction.[33]

Thus, although a genetic defect is the probable underlying etiology for CCHS when associated with HSCR, the probability for a successful search for candidate gene(s) accounting for the majority of CCHS cases appears relatively low at this time.

Animal Models

A true animal model displaying all or most of the phenotypic expression patterns of CCHS is not yet available. Schläfke and colleagues have demonstrated that after either electrocoagulation- or ibotenic acid-induced lesions of the intermediate area within the ventral medullary surface, significant compromise of both hypoxic and hypercapnic ventilatory responses will occur in anesthetized and awake cats.[34-36] Thus, this experimental model shares some of the typical respiratory control alterations found in CCHS patients (see below).

Despite the aforementioned negative genetic findings, several investigators have explored the possibility that genetic manipulation of the RET protooncogene in the mouse may lead to respiratory manifestations reminiscent of CCHS.[37] Indeed, markedly reduced ventilatory responses to hypercapnia were present in RET knock-out mice.[37] However, similar results were reported by Erickson et al. in brain-derived growth factor knock-out mice,[38] thereby suggesting that multiple genes may be involved in the regulation and development of respiratory control sites during embryogenesis.

Structural Central Nervous System Abnormalities

Based on the initial premise that a centrally-located defect is present in CCHS, it is not surprising that multiple attempts, albeit unsuccessful, have been made over the years to identify structural central nervous system abnormalities. Early reports of hypoplasia of the arcuate nucleus in one patient with CCHS,[39] and the presence of abnormal evoked potential responses to auditory stimuli[40-42] further suggested that a brainstem lesion may be present. In addition, central hypoventilation syndrome has been reported in occasional patients with cerebrovascular malformations,[43-47] and in patients with central nervous system infections.[48,49] However, a careful radiological survey of the brain in several CCHS patients has failed to identify a recognizable lesion accountable for the unique manifestations of this syndrome.[50]

More recently, using noninvasive functional MRI approaches which provide functional topographic maps of the brain in response to the application of specific stimulation paradigms,[51-55] we have shown disparate activation patterns of brainstem sites in 2 children with CCHS undergoing an hypercapnic challenge.[56] Indeed, in one CCHS child, no activation of ventromedullary and pontine sites occurred during 5% CO_2 breathing, while in the other CCHS patient, the extent and location of neural sites undergoing neuronal activity increases was similar to two age- and gender-matched controls.[56] Thus, these preliminary findings further add to the concept that CCHS is a very heterogeneous group of patients.

Clinical Presentation

Before undertaking the description of the physiological abnormalities present in older patients with CCHS, it is important to emphasize that the clinical presentation of CCHS may be quite variable and dependent on the severity of the disorder.[8] Some infants will not breathe at birth, and will require assisted ventilation in the newborn nursery. Most infants with CCHS who present in this manner do not breathe spontaneously during the first few months of life, but may mature to a pattern of adequate breathing during wakefulness over time. However, apnea or hypoventilation will persist during sleep. It is currently thought that this apparent improvement over the first few months of life results from normal maturation of the respiratory system, and does not represent a true change in the basic disorder.[57] Other infants may present at a later age with cyanosis, edema, and signs of right heart failure as the first indications of CCHS.[8] These infants have often been mistaken for cyanotic congenital heart disease patients. However, cardiac catheterization reveals only pulmonary hypertension. Infants with even less severe CCHS may present with tachycardia, diaphoresis, and/or cyanosis during sleep. Presumably, these infants will develop right heart failure as a consequence of repeated hypoxemic episodes during sleep if the diagnosis is not made. Still others may present with unexplained apnea, or an apparent life threatening event.[8]

Physiologic Abnormalities of Ventilatory Control

Wakefulness
Identification of the putative site inherent to CCHS manifestations could not only guide to better therapeutic approaches in these patients, but also provide extremely important insights onto modeling and localization of structures mediating respiratory control.

CCHS was initially considered to be a disorder of central chemoreceptor responsiveness only.[1-6] However, peripheral chemoreceptor pathways were not specifically tested. Paton and coworkers studied rebreathing hypoxic and hypercapnic ventilatory responses during wakefulness in 5 children with CCHS aged 6 - 11 years.[57] To measure the hypercapnic ventilatory response, children rebreathed a hyperoxic hypercapnic gas mixture until P_ACO_2 reached 56 - 69 torr, while for the hypoxic ventilatory response, children rebreathed a hypoxic gas mixture, at mixed venous PCO_2, until oxygen saturation (SPO_2) fell to $< 78\%$. In CCHS, ventilatory responses to both hypoxia and hypercapnia were essentially random, with no evidence of progressive ventilatory increases despite increasing stimulus. Paton and coworkers concluded that children with CCHS have absent chemoreceptor responses to both hypercapnia and hypoxia while awake.[57] They also speculated that the defect in CCHS may lie in the *central integration* of chemoreceptor signals.[57]

However, despite absent rebreathing ventilatory responses to both hypercapnia and hypoxia,[57] most CCHS patients are able to sustain adequate ventilation during wakefulness.[58] We hypothesized that the ability of CCHS patients to maintain waking ventilation could be related to either intact or residual peripheral chemoreceptor function.[59] To test this hypothesis, peripheral chemoreceptor response was assessed in 5 children with CCHS (ages 9 - 14 years) by measuring the ventilatory responses to 100% oxygen breathing, 5 tidal breaths of 100% N_2, and vital capacity breaths of 5% and 15% CO_2 in O_2 and 5% CO_2 in N_2. Tidal breathing of 100% O_2 resulted in similar ventilatory decreases in CCHS and matched controls. Acute hypoxia by N_2 tidal breathing resulted in a greater increase in respiratory rate in CCHS than in controls, but overall similar $\dot{V}_I$ increases. Vital capacity breaths of each of the CO_2-containing gas mixtures induced similar increases in $\dot{V}_I$ in CCHS and controls. The changes in $\dot{V}_I$ obtained with 15% CO_2 in O_2 and with 5% CO_2 in N_2 were significantly greater than those elicited by 5% CO_2 in O_2 suggesting a dose dependent response as well as additive effects of hypercapnic and hypoxic stimuli at the peripheral chemoreceptor level. Interestingly, for all responses a significantly greater coefficient of variation was found in CCHS patients. We concluded that peripheral chemoreceptor function, when assessed by acute hypoxia, hyperoxia or hypercapnia, was present and intact in CCHS children who were able to sustain adequate ventilation during wakefulness.[59] It is possible that the large interindividual variability of responses in CCHS may result from the lack of modulation of ventilatory control from either absent central chemoreceptor function and/or *defective integration* of afferent respiratory neural input.[59-60]

Since chemoreceptors are considered to be important controllers of ventilation during exercise, Paton et al. studied 5 CCHS children during an incremental exercise test on a treadmill.[61] At maximal exercise, oxygen uptake ($\dot{V}O_2$), and minute ventilation ($\dot{V}_I$) were lower in CCHS, but not significantly different from controls.[61] Compared to control children, CCHS increased $\dot{V}_I$ primarily by increasing respiratory frequency (f) rather than tidal volume (V_T). Furthermore, f and $\dot{V}_I$ increased proportionately to running frequency in CCHS (r = 0.88), suggesting preferential respiratory entrainment. SPO_2 fell, and $P_{ET}CO_2$ rose at maximal exercise in CCHS, but not in controls. Paton and coworkers concluded that exercise-induced hyperpnea can occur in the absence of chemoreceptor function.[61] They also speculated that, in the absence of ventilatory response to gradual chemoreceptor stimulation, movement exerts a dominant influence on respiratory rate, and consequently on minute ventilation during exercise.[61] Similar results showing significant alveolar hypoventilation in exercising CCHS and especially occurring at exercise loads above the anaerobic threshold have also been reported by other laboratories, further strengthening the concept that *central integration* of metabolic inputs is faulty in CCHS.[60,62]

We further hypothesized that rhythmic entrainment of respiration may contribute to $\dot{V}_I$ increases during exercise in CCHS.[63] To test the effect of motion on $\dot{V}_I$ in CCHS, we studied 6 CCHS patients during passive lower extremity motion at various frequencies. To achieve passive leg motion, subjects' feet were strapped to the pedals of a motorized cycle ergometer. Pedal frequency could be set from 6 to 60 RPM. The pedal motion was reversed to reduce the tendency for active pedaling. $\dot{V}_I$ was constant at pedal frequency 0 to 30 RPM, but increased significantly at pedal frequency $\geq$ 40 RPM in both controls and CCHS (*P* <

0.005). Respiratory rate and V_T increased similarly in both groups. However, $\dot{V}O_2$ was mildly increased at 60 RPM in both groups, suggesting some active muscular metabolic contribution at this pedaling rate to the primarily passive motion. $\dot{V}_I/\dot{V}O_2$ increased at pedal frequency 60 in CCHS, but remained constant in controls ($P < 0.03$). Similarly, $\dot{V}_I/\dot{V}O_2$ increased at pedal frequency 60 in CCHS, but remained constant in controls ($P < 0.04$). From pedal frequency 0 - 60, $P_{ET}CO_2$ decreased from 47 ± 7 to 41 ± 6 torr in CCHS ($P < 0.001$), but did not change in controls (38 ± 3 torr; NS). Heart rates increased similarly, and SPO_2 did not change in either group. It was concluded that passive leg motion at pedal frequency ≥ 40 will increase $\dot{V}_I$ in both CCHS and controls.[63] In controls, the increase in $\dot{V}_I$ was tightly coupled to the increase in $\dot{V}O_2$. However, in CCHS, passive leg motion elicited relative hyperventilation in excess of metabolic requirements, resulting in normalization of $P_{ET}CO_2$.[63] Thus, in a setting of deficient integration of respiratory control inputs, either mechanoreceptor afferent input from muscle and joints and/or rhythmic entrainment of respiration take over, and play a significant role in the modulation of breathing during exercise in children with CCHS.[63] Furthermore, normalization of $P_{ET}CO_2$ with motion as measured in CCHS would lend support to a basic defect in *integration* of efferent and afferent neural inputs to respiratory controllers sites.

Sleep
States of alertness exert profound influences on cardiorespiratory control. Respiratory output is primarily controlled by metabolic inputs during non-rapid eye movements (NREM) sleep. In contrast, during rapid eye movement (REM) sleep, the predominant control is not metabolic, but rather some form of "behavioral-like" drive, especially during phasic REM sleep.[64] CCHS is characterized by dysfunction in the metabolic control of breathing, such that the more severe gas exchange disturbances will occur during NREM sleep.[1-6,14] A recent study by Gaultier and colleagues demonstrated that while alveolar hypoventilation was particularly prominent during NREM sleep, hypercapnic chemosensitivity was unaffected by sleep states.[65] These data suggest that the intrinsic defect in CCHS is present at all times, but becomes more prominently expressed during conditions in which other redundant mechanisms are either less active or inoperative. Because ventilatory and arousal responses to respiratory stimuli may at least partially involve separate neural pathways, if CCHS children have a disorder of chemoreceptor input integration, they may still arouse to respiratory stimuli. To examine this issue, Marcus and colleagues performed hypercapnic arousal responses in 8 children with CCHS.[66] Children were studied during quiet sleep while normal ventilation was maintained using their home ventilators. For hypercapnic arousal responses, the P_ICO_2 was increased rapidly to 60 mmHg, and maintained until the child aroused or for a maximum duration of 3 minutes. Six of 8 (75%) CCHS children aroused to hypercapnia, and one additional child developed tachycardia (> 200) during hypercapnia. Marcus and coworkers concluded that most children with CCHS arouse to hypercapnia, indicating *intact* central chemoreceptor sensitivity.[66] They also speculated that because these children respond to hypercapnia, the most probable mechanism for CCHS is a brainstem lesion in the area where input from chemoreceptors is *integrated*.[66]

Autonomic Nervous System Dysfunction

As mentioned above, CCHS is characterized by abnormal ventilatory control in the absence of obvious anatomic lesions. Woo et al. hypothesized that CCHS patients may also have disturbances in autonomic nervous system function.[67] To test this, they measured moment-to-moment heart rate variability in 12 patients with CCHS and in age- and sex-matched controls using standard deviation of R-R intervals, R-R interval spectral analysis, and Poincaré plots of sequential R-R intervals (R-R$_n$ *versus* R-R$_{n+1}$) over a 24-hour period using ambulatory Holter monitoring.[67] Sleep and wakefulness were determined from subjects' diaries. Mean heart rates in CCHS and controls were similar. Standard deviation analysis of R-R intervals also showed similar results in both groups. Using spectral analysis, the LOW-HIGH frequency spectra ratios decreased in sleep compared to wakefulness in all controls. During wakefulness, the LOW-HIGH ratios were similar in both CCHS and controls. However, an increase in the LOW-HIGH ratio was observed during sleep compared to wakefulness in 11 of 12 CCHS ($P < 0.001$). Poincaré plots displayed significantly reduced beat-to-beat interval changes at slower heart rates in the CCHS patients. The patterns of points in CCHS Poincaré plots were easily distinguished from the patterns in controls by seven blinded observers. Woo and coworkers concluded that all CCHS patients showed disturbed moment-to-moment heart rate variability.[67] They also speculated that these changes suggest that CCHS patients exhibit alterations in autonomic nervous system control of the heart, which in turn could indicate widespread dysfunction of autonomic *integration*.[67] These findings have been further corroborated by a later independent study of CCHS patients,[68] and have even been identified pre-natally in an infant diagnosed with CCHS after birth.[69]

Significant alterations in dopamine turnover were found in patients with CCHS,[70] and vagally-mediated syncope may also occur in CCHS children [71, Gozal D: personal communication], thereby lending further support to the assumption that significant dysregulation of central autonomic nervous system control is frequently present in CCHS.

Summary

Awareness to the existence of CCHS has led to increasingly frequent reports of such patients from all over the world. However, the pathophysiologal mechanisms underlying the clinical manifestations of this congenital disease entity remain unknown. For the respiratory physiologist, CCHS can be viewed as an experiment of nature which provides an important and unique window into central cardiorespiratory regulation. For the pediatrician, CCHS children represent an unique clinical challenge in the search for the right combination between technological advances and quality of life.

The author is supported in part by grants from the National Institute of Health (HD-01072), the Maternal and Child Health Bureau (MCJ-229163), and the American Lung Association (CI-002-N).

References

1. Mellins RB, Balfour HH Jr, Turino GM, Winters RW. Failure of automatic control of ventilation (Ondine's curse). *Medicine* 49: 487-504, 1970.

2. Fishman LS, Samson JH, Sperling DR. Primary alveolar hypoventilation syndrome (Ondine's curse). *Amer J Dis Child* 110: 155-161, 1965.

3. Deonna T, Arczynska W, Torrado A. Congenital failure of automatic ventilation (Ondine's curse). *J Pediatr* 84: 710-714, 1974.

4. Shannon DC, Marsland DW, Gould JB, Callahan B, Todres ID, Dennis J. Central hypoventilation during quiet sleep in two infants. *Pediatrics* 57: 342-346, 1976.

5. Fleming PJ, Cade D, Bryan MH, Bryan AC. Congenital central hypoventilation and sleep state. *Pediatrics* 66: 425-428, 1980.

6. Guilleminault C, McQuitty J, Ariagno RL, Challamel MJ, Korobkin R, McClead RE. Congenital central alveolar hypoventilation syndrome in six infants. *Pediatrics* 70: 684-694, 1982.

7. Oren J, Kelly DH, Shannon DC. Long-term follow-up of children with congenital central hypoventilation syndrome. *Pediatrics* 80: 375-380, 1987.

8. Marcus CL, Jansen MT, Poulsen MK, Keens SE, Nield TA, Lipsker LE, Keens TG. Medical and psychosocial outcome of children with congenital central hypoventilation syndrome. *J Pediatr* 119: 888-895, 1991.

9. Weese-Mayer DE, Silvestri JM, Menzies LJ, Morrow-Kenny AS, Hunt CE, Hauptman SA. Congenital central hypoventilation syndrome: diagnosis, management, and long-term outcome in thirty-two children. *J Pediatr* 120: 381-387, 1992.

10. Keens, T., and T. Hoppenbrouwers. Congenital central hypoventilation syndrome (770.81). In: *Diagnostic Classification Steering Committee of the American Sleep Disorders Association. The International Classification of Sleep Disorders: Diagnostic and Coding Manual*. Allen Press Inc, Lawrence, Kansas, pp 205-209, 1990.

11. Severinghaus JW, Mitchell RA. Ondine's Curse: Failure of respiratory center automaticity while awake. *Clin Res* 10: 122, 1962.

12 Hunt CE, Matalon SV, Thompson TT. Central hypoventilation syndrome: experience with bilateral phrenic nerve pacing in 3 neonates. *Am Rev Respir Dis* 118: 23-28, 1978.

13. Wells HH, Kattwinkel J, Morrow ID. Control of ventilation in Ondine's curse. *J Pediatr* 96: 865-867, 1980.

14 Haddad GG, Mazza NM, Defendini R, Blanc WA, Driscoll JM, Epstein AF, Epstein RA,. Mellins RB. Congenital failure of automatic control of ventilation, gastrointestinal motility and heart rate. *Medicine* 57: 517-526, 1978.

15. Weese-Mayer DE, Silvestri JM, Marazita ML, Hoo JJ. Congenital central hypoventilation syndrome: inheritance and relation to sudden infant death syndrome. *Am J Med Genet* 47: 360-367, 1993.

16. Khalifa MM, Flavin MA, Wherrett BA. Congenital central hypoventilation syndrome in monozygotic twins. *J Pediatr* 113: 853-855, 1988.

17. Minutillo C, Pemberton PJ, Goldblatt J. Hirschsprung's disease and Ondine's curse: further evidence for a distinct syndrome. *Clin Genet* 36: 200-203, 1989.

18. Nakahara S, Yokomori K, Tamura K, Oku K, Tsuchida Y. Hirschsprung's disease associated with Ondine's curse: a special subgroup? *J Pediatr Surg* 10 : 1481-1484, 1995.

19. el-Halaby E, Coran AG. Hirschsprung's disease associated with Ondine's curse: report of three cases and review of the literature. *J Pediatr Surg* 29: 530-535, 1994.

20. Fodstad H, Ljunggren B, Shawis R. Ondine's curse with Hirschsprung's disease. *Br J Neurosurg* 4: 87-93, 1990.

21. Verloes A, Elmer C, Lacombe D, Heinrichs C, Rebuffat E, Demarquez JL, Moncla A, Adam E. Ondine-Hirschsprung syndrome (Haddad syndrome). Further delineation in two cases and

review of the literature. *Eur J Pediatr* 152: 75-77, 1993.

22. Edery P, Lyonnet S, Mulligan LM, Pelet A, Dow E, Abel L, Holder S, Nihoul-Fekete C, Ponder BA, Munnich A. Mutations of the RET proto-oncogene in Hirschsprung's disease. *Nature* 367: 378-380, 1994.

23. Romeo G, Ronchetto P, Luo Y, Barone V, Seri M, Ceccherini I, Pasini B, Bocciardi R, Lerone M, Kaariainen H. Point mutations affecting the tyrosine kinase domain of the RET proto-oncogene in Hirschsprung's disease. *Nature* 367: 377-378, 1994.

24. Schuchardt A, D'Agati V, Larsson-Blomberg L, Costantini F, Pachnis V. Defects in the kidney and enteric nervous system of mice lacking the tyrosine kinase receptor Ret. *Nature* 367: 380-383, 1994.

25. Swaminathan S, Gilsanz V, Atkinson J, Keens TG. Congenital central hypoventilation syndrome associated with multiple ganglioneuromas. *Chest* 96: 423-424, 1989.

26. Poceta JS, Strandjord TP, Badura Jr RJ, Milstein JM. Ondine curse and neurocristopathy. *Pediatr Neurol* 6: 370-372, 1987.

27. Stovroff M, Dykes F, Teague WG. The complete spectrum of neurocristopathy in an infant with congenital hypoventilation, Hirschsprung's disease, and neuroblastoma. *J Pediatr Surg* 30: 1218-1221, 1995.

28. Roshkow JE, Haller JO, Berdon WE, Sane SM. Hirschsprung's disease, Ondine's curse, and neuroblastoma--manifestations of neurocristopathy. *Pediatr Radiol* 19: 45-49, 1988.

29. Amiel J, Attie T, Simeoni J, Edery P, Gaultier C, Munnich A, Lyonnet S. Mutation of the *ret* proto-oncogene in a patient with congenital central hypoventilation syndrome (Ondine's curse) and Hirschsprung disease. *Am J Human Gen* 57: A205, 1995.

30. Bolk S, Weese-Mayer DE, Silvestri JM, Chakravarti A. Congenital central hypoventilation syndrome: mutation analysis of the receptor tyrosine kinase RET. *Am J Med Genet* 63: 603-609, 1996.

31. Kinane TB, Burton MD. A genetic approach to the congenital central hypoventilation syndrome. *Pediatr Pulmonol* 23: 133-135, 1997.

32. Bolk S, Angrist M, Xie J, Yanagisawa M, Silvestri JM, Weese-Mayer DE, Chakravarti A. Endothelin-3 frameshift mutation in congenital central hypoventilation syndrome. *Nat Genet* 13: 395-396, 1996 (letter).

33. Marcus CL, Livingston FR, Wood SE, Keens TG. Hypercapnic and hypoxic ventilatory responses in parents and siblings of children with congenital central hypoventilation syndrome. *Am Rev Respir Dis* 144: 36-40, 1991.

34. Schläfke ME, Kille JF, Loeschcke HH. Elimination of central chemosensitivity by coagulation of a bilateral area on the ventral medullary surface in awake cats. *Pflüger Arch* 378: 231-241, 1979.

35. Schläfke ME, See WR, Herker-See A, Loeschke HH. Respiratory response to hypoxia and hypercapnia after elimination of central chemosensitivity. *Pflüger Arch* 381: 241-248, 1979.

36. Schafer D, Schläfke ME. Cardiorespiratory regulation in a model for Ondine's curse syndrome. In: *Ventral Brainstem Mechanisms and Control of Respiration and Blood Bressure.* Edited by Trouth OC, Millis RM, Kiwull-Schöne HF, Schläfke ME. Marcel Dekker Inc, pp 675-685, 1995.

37. Burton MS, Kawashima A, Brayer JA, Kazemi H, Shannon DC, Schuchardt A, Costantini F, Pachnis V, Kinane TB. RET proto-oncogene is important for the development of respiratory CO_2 sensitivity. *J Auton Nerv Syst* 63: 137-143, 1997.

38. Erickson JT, Conover JC, Borday V, Champagnat J, Barbacid M, Yancopoulos G, Katz DM. Mice lacking brain-derived neurotrophic factor exhibit visceral sensory neuron losses distinct

from mice lacking NT4 and display a severe developmental deficit in control of breathing. *J Neurosci* 16: 5361-5371, 1996.

39. Folgering H, Kuyper F, Kille JF. Primary alveolar hypoventilation (Ondine s curse syndrome) in an infant without external arcuate nucleus. Case Report. *Bull Eur Physiopathol Respir* 15: 659-665, 1979.

40. Long KJ, Allen N. Abnormal brain-stem auditory evoked potentials following Ondine's curse. *Arch Neurol* 41: 1109-1110, 1984.

41. Litscher G, Schwarz G, Reimann R. Abnormal brain stem auditory evoked potentials in a girl with the central alveolar hypoventilation syndrome. *Int J Neurosci* 87: 113-117, 1996.

42. Beckerman RC, Meltzer J, Sola A, Dunn D, Weggman M. Brainstem auditory response in Ondine's syndrome. *Arch Neurol* 43: 698-701, 1986.

43. Cutz E, Ma TKPerrin DG, Moore AM, Becker LE. Peripheral chemoreceptors in congenital central hypoventilation syndrome. *Am J Respir Crit Care Med* 155: 358-363, 1997.

44. Mukhopadhyay S, Wilkinson PW. Cerebral arteriovenous malformation, Ondine's curse and Hirschsprung's disease. *Dev Med Child Neurol* 32: 1087-1089, 1990.

45. Beal MF, Richardson Jr. EP, Brandstetter R, Hedley-Whyte ET, Hochberg FH. Localized brainstem ischemic damage and Ondine's curse after near-drowning. *Neurology* 33: 717-721, 1983.

46. Bogousslavsky J, Khurana R, Deruaz JP, Hornung JP, Regli F, Janzer R, Perret C. Respiratory failure and unilateral caudal brainstem infarction. *Ann Neurol* 28: 668-673, 1990.

47. Liu HM, Loew JM, Hunt CE. Congenital central hypoventilation syndrome: a pathologic study of the neuromuscular system. *Neurology* 28: 1013-1019, 1978.

48. Jensen TH, Hansen PB, Brodersen P. Ondine's curse in listeria monocytogenes brain stem encephalitis. *Acta Neurol Scand* 77: 505-506, 1988.

49. Giangaspero F, Schiavina M, Sturani C, Mondini S, Cirignotta F. Failure of automatic control of ventilation (Ondine's curse) associated with viral encephalitis of the brainstem: a clinicopathologic study of one case. *Clin Neuropathol* 7: 234-237, 1988.

50. Weese Mayer DE, Brouillette RT, Naidich TP, McClone DG, Hunt CE. Magnetic resonance imaging and computerized tomography in central hypoventilation. *Am Rev Respir Dis* 137: 393-398, 1988.

51. Ogawa S, Lee TM, Nayak AS, Glynn P. Oxygenation-sensitive contrast in magnetic resonance image of rodent brain at high magnetic fields. *Magnet Reson Med* 14: 68-78, 1990.

52. Hathout GM, Gambhir SS, Gopi RK, Kirlew KAT, Choi Y, So G, Gozal D, Harper RM, Lufkin RB, Hawkins R. A quantitative physiologic model of blood oxygenation for functional magnetic resonance imaging. *Invest Radiol* 30: 669-682, 1995.

53. Gozal D, Hathout GM, Kirlew KAT, Tang H, Woo MS, Zhang J, Lufkin RB, Harper RM. Localization of putative neural respiratory regions in the human by functional magnetic resonance imaging. *J Appl Physiol* 76: 2076-2083, 1994.

54. Gozal D, Omidvar O, Kirlew KAT, Hathout GM, Hamilton R, Lufkin RB, Harper RM. Identification of human brain regions underlying responses to inspiratory loading with functional magnetic resonance imaging. *Proc Nat Acad Sci USA* 92: 6607-6611, 1995.

55. Gozal D, Omidvar O, Kirlew KAT, Hathout GM, Lufkin RB, Harper RM. Brain regions mediating the response to resistive expiratory loads in humans. *J Clin Invest* 97: 47-53, 1996.

56. Gozal D. Novel functional imaging strategies in assessment of respiratory control. *Pediatr Pulmonol* 23: 148-150, 1997.

57. Paton JY, Swaminathan S, Sargent CW, Keens TG. Hypoxic and hypercapneic ventilatory responses in awake children with congenital central hypoventilation syndrome. *Amer Rev*

Respir Dis 140: 368-372, 1989.

58. Shea SA, Andres LP, Paydarfar A, Banzett RB, Shannon DC. Effect of mental activity on breathing in congenital central hypoventilation syndrome. *Respir Physiol* 94: 251-263, 1993.

59. Gozal D, Marcus CL, Shoseyov D, Keens TG. Peripheral chemoreceptor function in children with congenital central hypoventilation syndrome. *J Appl Physiol,* 74: 379-387, 1993.

60. Shea SA, Andres LP, Shannon DC, Banzett RB. Ventilatory responses to exercise in humans lacking ventilatory chemosensitivity. *J Physiol (Lond)* 468: 623-640, 1993.

61. Paton JY, Swaminathan S, Sargent CW, Hawksworth A, Keens TG. Ventilatory response to exercise in children with congenital central hypoventilation syndrome. *Am Rev Resp Dis* 147: 1185-1191, 1993.

62. Silvestri JM, Weese-Mayer DE, Flanagan EA. Congenital central hypoventilation syndrome: cardiorespiratory responses to moderate exercise, simulating daily activity. *Pediatr Pulmonol* 20: 89-93, 1995.

63. Gozal D, Marcus CL, Davidson Ward SL, Keens TG. Ventilatory responses to passive leg motion in children with Congenital Central Hypoventilation Syndrome. *Am J Resp Crit Care Med* 153: 761-768, 1996.

64. Phillipson EA, Bowes G. Control of breathing during sleep. In: *Handbook of Physiology: The Respiratory System, vol 2.* Edited by Cherniack NS and Widdicombe JG. Bethesda, MD, USA, American Physiological Society, pp 649-689, 1986.

65. Gaultier C, Trang-Pham H, Praud JP, Gallego J. Cardiorespiratory control during sleep in the congenital central hypoventilation syndrome. *Pediatr Pulmonol* 23: 140-142, 1997.

66. Marcus CL, Bautista DB, Amihyia A, Davidson Ward SL, Keens TG. Hypercapneic arousal responses in children with congenital central hypoventilation syndrome. *Pediatrics* 88: 993-998, 1991.

67. Woo MS, Woo MA, Gozal D, Jansen MT, Keens TG, Harper RM. Heart rate variability in congenital central hypoventilation syndrome. *Pediatr Res* 31: 291-296, 1992.

68. Ogawa T, Kojo M, Fukushima N, Sonoda H, Goto K, Ishiwa S, Ishiguro M. Cardio-respiratory control in an infant with Ondine's curse: a multivariate autoregressive modelling approach. *J Auton Nerv Syst* 42: 41-52, 1993.

69. Lang U, Braems G, Kunzel W. Heart rate alterations in a fetus with Ondine's curse. *Gynecol Obstet Invest* 30: 124 - 126, 1990.

70. Hedner J, Hedner T, Breese GR, Lundell KH, Lundberg D, Lundstrom NR, Ostergaard E, McCown TJ, Mueller RA. Changes in cerebrospinal fluid homovanillic acid in children with Ondine's curse. *Pediatr Pulmonol* 3: 131-135, 1987.

71. O'Sullivan J, Cottrell AJ, Wren C. Ondine's curse and neurally mediated syncope-a new and important association. *Eur Heart J* 14: 1289-1291, 1993.

Alternating versus synchronous ventilation of the two lungs

Adrian Versprille and Jos R.C. Jansen

Independent ventilation of each lung was performed in 1972 by Seed and Sykes[1] using a tracheal divider. They called this technique differential ventilation (DV). Subsequently, DV has been used to apply different ventilatory patterns to each lung in patients with predominantly unilateral lung disease (references before 1983,[2] later[3-5]). DV, applied either synchronously (SV) or non-synchronously,[6,7] did not decrease cardiac output when compared to conventional, common ventilation of both lungs. Alternating ventilation, in which one lung is inflated while the other is being deflated, was applied by Muneyuki et al. in 1983 in mongrel dogs.[8] They observed no changes in cardiac output between synchronous and alternating ventilation (AV) in spite of a significant decrease in oesophageal pressure, as a substitute for intrathoracic pressure. We reasoned that during AV, volume expansion of one lung by inflation would cause an expiration of the opposite lung below its end-expiratory volume as existing during SV, due to compression. Consequently, its mean volume and therefore mean thoracic expansion (and intrathoracic pressure) would be less during AV than during SV, causing a lower central venous pressure.

We hypothesized that alternating ventilation (AV) to each lung would reduce mean central venous pressure resulting in an increased cardiac output. In three successive studies[9-11] we tested this hypothesis in anaesthetized piglets. AV was applied after insertion of an endobronchial tube into the main left bronchus, via a branch of a Y-shaped tracheal cannula. The other branch was used to ventilate the right lung. The technique of differential ventilation, insertion and air tight positioning of the endobronchial tube is described in detail in the mentioned papers. The technique of insertion of the endobronchial tube is simple and easy to perform without disturbance of the steady state conditions of the animals. In Fig. 1 the modes of SV and AV are shown.

In the first study[9] we ventilated right and left lung by subdividing the normal tidal volume (V_T) into tidal volumes to the left ($V_{T,l}$) and the right lung ($V_{T,r}$) respectively, on guidance of an equal left and right airway pressure. These pressures were also equal to the airway pressure during the preceding phase of common ventilation: thus, $P_{aw,r} = P_{aw,l} = P_{aw}$. From the three studies we obtained a value for $V_{T,r} / V_{T,l} = 1.24 \pm 0.10$ in 20 pigs. Thus, total ventilation during AV was equal to that during common ventilation, which was adapted to normocapnic conditions. These conditions were not changed by AV, also arterial oxygenation was maintained during AV.

We found a decrease in central venous pressure and an increase in cardiac output during AV compared to SV under conditions of the same minute ventilation (table 1). Furthermore, pulmonary arterial pressure (P_{pa}) was slightly but significantly increased, which we ascribed to the increased cardiac output. Heart rate did not change, physiological dead space decreased and venous admixture increased a little.

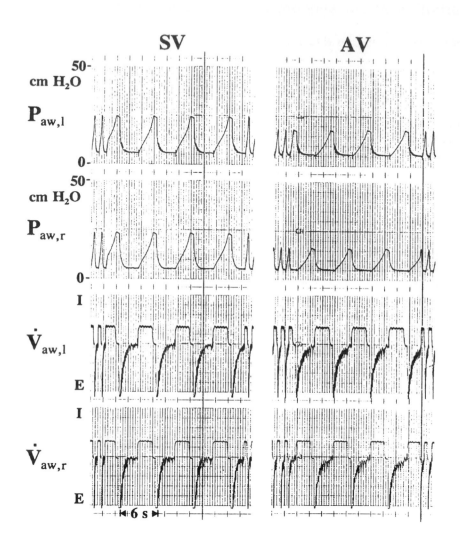

Figure 1. An individual example of synchronous (SV), left panel, and alternating ventilation (AV), right panel. $P_{aw,l}$ and $P_{aw,r}$: left and right airway pressures, measured in the endobronchial tube and the tracheal cannula respectively; $V'_{aw,l}$ and $V'_{aw,r}$: air flow measured in the tubes connecting ventilators and endobronchial tube and tracheal cannula respectively. I and E are inspiratory and expiratory flow. Inflation phase of one lung is half a ventilatory cycle out of phase with the inflation of the other lung. During AV peak and pause airway pressures are lower compared to those during SV. Obtained from ref. 10 with courtesy of Intensive Care Medicine.

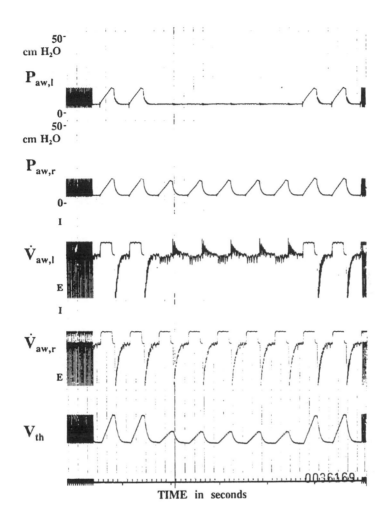

Figure 2. Individual example of right-to-left cross talk between both lungs. Symbols as in Fig.1. V_{th}: recording of the mercury-in-rubber cord signal around the thorax, where an upwards flection represents thorax expansion in arbitrary units. These units were calibrated by inflation of known volumes to analyze lung volume changes off line from computer recordings.

Cross-talk: inflation of the right lung coincided with an expiratory flow from the left lung and expiration of the right lung with a spontaneous, inspiratory flow into the left lung. The expiratory and inspiratory flow signals of the left lung were integrated separately. The zero-line for these integrations was determined as the virtual horizontal line through the moment of zero flow at the end of the inspiratory pause, immediately before the expiration, as observed during ventilation of the left lung before and after the period of unilateral ventilation. Obtained from ref. 11 with courtesy of Intensive Care Medicine.

We explained the higher cardiac output during AV compared to SV by the decrease in central venous pressure according to the theory of Guyton on venous return,[12, 13] which we confirmed for conditions of intact circulation.[14] The decrease in mean central venous pressure was ascribed to a decrease in intrathoracic pressure, which we hypothetically based on a compression of the heterolateral lung during one-sided inflation. As a consequence a lower mean lung volume and, therefore, a lower mean intrathoracic volume and mean intrathoracic pressure would occur during alternating inflation of the two lungs.

In the second study[10] we obtained evidence for the decrease in intrathoracic pressure. In a first series of observations oesophageal pressure and in a second series pericardial pressure was lower during AV than during SV. Again we found a higher cardiac output and aortic pressure and a lower central venous pressure during AV in a similar way as in the first study. Oesophageal and pericardial pressure were significantly reduced from 1.0 ± 1.4 mm Hg and 1.5 ± 1.1 mm Hg during SV to 0.6 ± 1.6 and 0.9 ± 1.0 mm Hg respectively during AV, P- values < 0.001.

Table 1. Haemodynamic and ventilatory data during alternating and simultaneous ventilation

	AV		SV		Difference		
	Mean	SD	Mean	SD	Mean	SD	P-value
Q'_T	2.07	0.32	1.88	0.30	0.19	0.09	< 0.001
P_{cv}	1.8	1.1	2.4	1.3	−0.66	0.31	< 0.001
P_{ao}	101	7	96	7	64	3.7	< 0.001
P_{pa}	13.8	2.2	14.4	2.0	−0.52	0.60	$= 0.001$
Q'_s/Q'_T	4.8	3.3	4.5	3.2	0.37	0.45	< 0.001
F_H	150	26	148	26	2.5	0.34	
V_D/V_T	32.0	4.0	34.2	3.7	−2.2	2.1	< 0.001

AV: alternating ventilation; SV: simultaneous ventilation; Difference: differences between the variables during AV and SV. Mean: mean of all individual data; SD: ± standard deviation; P-value, calculated with use of a paired T-test for the differences; 3 observations per pig, i.e. n = 21. Q'_T (ml $s^{-1}kg^{-1}$): cardiac output, determined with the Fick method; P_{cv} (mm Hg): central venous pressure; P_{ao} (mm Hg): aortic pressure; P_{pa} (mm Hg): pulmonary artery pressure; Q'_s/Q'_T (% of Q'_T): venous admixture or right-to-left shunt in the pulmonary circulation; F_H (beats/min): heart rate; V_D/V_T (% of V_T): physiological dead space. Data obtained from ref. 9 by courtesy of Intensive Care Medicine.

In our third study we tested the hypothesis that the opposite lung would be compressed during one-sided lung inflation as a reason for the lower intrathoracic pressure. During SV we inserted periods of unilateral ventilation of either the left or right lung during five ventilatory cycles. During inflation and expiration of the ventilated lung we observed an expiratory and inspiratory flow respectively from and into the opposite, non-ventilated lung (fig. 2). We called this phenomenon of interaction cross-talk between the lungs. The expired flow indicated a volume loss from the opposite lung. Volume compression was determined from integrating the outflow pattern from the non-inflated lung during inflation of the other lung. Because we found a $V_{T,r}$ / $V_{T,l}$ > 1 in all pigs, we concluded that the volume of the right lung was larger than that of the left lung. In twenty pigs, the amount of compression of the right lung was 1.55 ± 0.43 ml/kg body weight (mean $\pm$ SD), caused by a tidal volume to the left lung of 7.33 ± 1.06 ml/kg, i.e. a compression of the right lung of 21 ± 4.5 % of the left tidal volume. The left lung compression was 1.34 ± 0.41 ml/kg caused by $V_{T,r} = 9.07 \pm 1.21$ ml/kg, implying a compression of the left lung equal to 15 ± 3.9 % of $V_{T,r}$. Thus, a smaller inflation into the smaller left lung compressed the larger right lung more than a larger inflation into the larger right lung did on the smaller left lung.

We have no explanation for the larger left-to-right cross-talk than r-to-l cross-talk, which is undoubtedly due to a lack of understanding how the cross-talk will occur. A transmediastinal way might occur, but also a route via an increase in abdominal pressure, acting on the volume of the non-inflated lung might be possible. Furthermore, some effect of a shift in perfusion from the inflated to the non-ventilated lung could contribute. However, each of the pathways will not a priori imply an explanation of the mentioned difference between the l-to-r and r-to-l cross-talk. Then, additional quantitative analyses will be needed.

References
1. Seed RF, Sykes MK. Differential lung ventilation. *Brit J Anaesthesiol* 44: 758-765, 1972.
2. Geiger K. Differential Lung ventilation. In: *European Advances in Intensive Care*. Edited by Geiger K. Little, Brown and Company, Boston, 21: 83-96, 1983.
3. Baerentz S, Hedenstierna G. Differential ventilation and selective positive end-expiratory pressure: effects on patients with acute bilateral lung disease. *Anesthesiology* 61: 511-517, 1984.
4. Klingstedt C, Hedenstierna G, Baehrendtz S, Lundquist H, Strandberg A, Tokics L, Brismar B. Ventilation-perfusion relationships and atelectasis formation in the supine and lateral positions during conventional mechanical and differential ventilation. *Acta Anaesthesiol Scand* 34: 421-429, 1990.
5. Klingstedt C, Hedenstierna G, Lundquist H, Tokics L, Brismar B. The influence of body position and differential ventilation on lung dimensions and atelectasis formation in anaesthesized man. *Acta Anaesthesiol Scand* 34: 315-322, 1990.
6. Frostell C, Hedenstierna G, Cronestrand R. Asynchronous ventilation in the dogs: effects on lung blood flow and gas exchange. *Clin Physiol* 5: Suppl 3: 59-64, 1985.
7. Hillman KM, Barber JD. Asynchronous independent lung ventilation (AILV). *Crit Care Med* 8: 390 - 395, 1980.
8. Muneyuki M, Konishi K, Horiguchi R, Tsujimoto S, Saito M, Sakakura S, Konishi A. Effects of alternating lung ventilation on cardiopulmonary functions in dogs. *Anesthesiol* 58: 353-356, 1983.
9. Versprille A, Hrachovina V, Jansen JRC. Alternating versus synchronous ventilation of left and right lungs in piglets. *Intensive Care Med* 21: 1009-1015, 1995.
10. Versprille A, Oosterhout M van, Jansen JRC. Haemodynamic and ventilatory responses on alternating ventilation of left and right lungs. *Intensive Care Med* 22: 813-817, 1996.
11. Versprille A, Oosterhout M. van. Cross-talk between the lungs in piglets. *Intensive Care Med* 22: 1082-1089, 1996.
12. Guyton AC, AW Lindsey, BN Kaufmann. Effect of mean circulatory filling pressure and other

peripheral circulatory factors on cardiac output. *Am J Physiol* 180: 463-468, 1955.
13. Guyton AC, CE Jones, TG Coleman. *Circulatory Physiology*: Cardiac Output and its Regulation. WB Saunders Company, Philadelphia, 1973.
14. Versprille A, JRC Jansen. Mean systemic filling pressure as a characteristic pressure for venous return. *Pflügers Arch* 405: 226-233, 1985.

(Endogenous) Opioids and the cardiovascular system

James G. Bovill

While modulation of nociception is often considered the primary effect of the endogenous opioid system, it has become clear during the past decade that this system exhibits a remarkable complexity, with functional implications for most organs, including the cardiovascular system. Endogenous opioid peptides and their receptors are present in brain areas responsible for cardiovascular control, in the heart, in autonomic ganglia and in the adrenal medulla, and influence and regulate cardiovascular functions both centrally and peripherally. They are involved in the modulation of hypertension and in other pathological cardiovascular conditions such as congestive heart failure and myocardial ischaemia. Endogenous opioid peptides are released upon myocardial ischaemia and contribute to the development of ischaemic arrhythmias and cardiogenic shock.[1-3] Some of these effects are reversed by the opioid antagonist, naloxone.[4] Dynorphin, the endogenous ligand for the κ-receptors, appears to be the most potent of the endogenous opioid peptides in the induction of cardiac arrhythmias.[2] The endogenous opioid peptides also appear to be involved in the pathogenesis of acute myocardial infarction.[5] Both δ- and κ-receptors are present in the heart,[6] and large amounts of mRNA for preproenkephalin A have been identified in ventricular myocytes of rats and hamsters, suggesting that cardiac myocytes are capable of synthesising opioid peptides.[7,8]

While κ-receptor agonists have no effect on cardiovascular function in healthy humans,[9] release of endogenous opioid peptides and activation of δ- and κ-receptors during congestive heart failure decreases myocardial mechanical performance and alters regional blood flow distribution.[3] Opioid receptor antagonists may exert beneficial cardiovascular effects in heart failure. Initially, the cardiovascular effects of the endogenous opioids was thought to be due exclusively to pre-synaptic mechanisms, i.e. to an opioid peptide modulation of neurotransmitter release from autonomic nerve terminals within the heart. With the recognition that opioid receptors and endogenous opioid peptides are present in the heart itself, it has been discovered that an important mechanism for the negative inotropic and other adverse cardiovascular effects is an elevation of intracellular free Ca^{2+} $[Ca^{2+}]_i$. This is due to an increased mobilization of calcium from intracellular stores subsequent upon an increased production of inositol-1,4,5-triphosphate (IP_3). The increase in $[Ca^{2+}]_i$ may manifest in cardiac arrhythmias while depletion of calcium from intracellular stores is responsible for a reduction in contractility.[3,10,11] Further there is an intimate relationship between opioid receptors and the β-adrenergic system within the heart.[12]

Until recently it was not known whether μ-opioid receptors were present in the heart. However, Saeki and colleagues[13] have demonstrated that these receptors are present in cardiac pacemaker cells in the rabbit. They found that fentanyl, a selective μ-opioid receptor agonist, decreased the action potential amplitude, maximum rate of depolarisation and spontaneous firing frequency and prolonged the action potential duration in a concentration-dependent manner in isolated strips of sinoatrial node. The concentrations of fentanyl producing these effects (0.1-3 µM) were comparable to those used during anaesthesia. The actions of fentanyl were completely blocked by β-funaltrexamine, an irreversible µ-receptor antagonist, but were not affected by selective δ- or κ-receptor antagonists, nor by pretreatment with atropine or propranolol. The negative chronotropic effect of fentanyl was due to a decrease in the conductance of all membrane currents and a decrease in the fast and slow components of the delayed rectifying K^+ current.

While the concentrations of endogenous opioid peptides are increased in patients with acute heart failure, the concentrations are decreased in patients with chronic heart failure.[14] This has been interpreted as exhaustion of the opioid system.[15] Morphine produced dose-related decreases in the contractility of atria obtained from non-failing and failing human hearts, but the concentration-response curve was significantly shifted to the right in preparations from failing hearts.[16] The negative inotropic effects induced by morphine in both failing and non-failing preparations were not antagonized by naloxone, indicating that opioid receptors do not play a part in this cardiac effect of morphine. One explanation could be an interaction with β-adrenoceptors, unrelated to the binding of opioids to opioid receptors. Opioids inhibit β-adrenoceptor-sensitive adenylyl cyclase.[17]

Most of the haemodynamic effects of opioid drugs in humans can be related to their reduction of sympathetic outflow from the CNS, specific vagal effects or, in the case of morphine and pethidine, histamine release. Fentanyl and its analogues do not cause histamine release.[18] Depression of baroreceptor reflexes by opioids may also contribute to the overall haemodynamic response. Fentanyl impairs the carotid chemoreceptor reflex, which is not only of importance in the control of respiration, but also acts as a powerful cardiovascular reflex.[19]

Fentanyl and sufentanil enhance the calcium current that occurs during the plateau phase (phase 2) of the cardiac action potential, and depress the outward potassium current responsible for terminal repolarisation,[20] resulting in a significant prolongation of the duration of the action potential. Blair et al.[21] suggested that the cardiac electrophysiological effects of fentanyl and sufentanil represented a direct membrane effect resembling that produced by class III anti-arrhythmic drugs. The anti-arrhythmic properties of some κ-receptor agonists may, however, be due to blockade of sodium channels (a class I effect), but this may be independent of any agonism at the κ-receptor, since it is not blocked by naloxone.[22] In patients, large doses of opioids prolong the QT interval of the ECG.[20] This may explain the reported anti-arrhythmic properties of opioids, particularly in the presence of myocardial ischaemia.[23] Fentanyl, 60 µg kg[-1], and sufentanil, 10 µg kg[-1], significantly increased the ventricular fibrillation threshold in dogs following coronary artery occlusion.[24]

All opioid drugs, with the exception of pethidine, produce bradycardia, although morphine given to healthy subjects may cause tachycardia. Pethidine often produces tachycardia, possibly due to the similarities in structure between it and atropine. The mechanism of opioid-induced bradycardia is central vagal stimulation. Premedication with atropine can minimize, but may not totally eliminate, opioid-induced bradycardia, especially in patients taking β-adrenoceptor antagonists. The speed of injection appears to be important, particularly with the more potent drugs; slow administration minimizing bradycardia. Although severe bradycardia should obviously be avoided, moderate slowing of HR is not harmful and, by reducing myocardial oxygen consumption, may be beneficial, especially in patients with coronary heart disease.

Isolated heart or heart-muscle studies have demonstrated dose-related negative inotropic effects for morphine, pethidine, fentanyl and alfentanil.[25-28] However, these effects occurred at concentrations one hundred to several thousand times those found clinically, even during high-dose opioid anaesthesia. In canine hearts the direct intra-coronary injection of fentanyl in concentrations up to 240 ng ml^{-1} produced no changes in myocardial mechanical function.[29] After a bolus intravenous dose of fentanyl, 75 to 100 μg kg^{-1}, peak plasma concentrations are seldom above 100 ng ml^{-1}, and fall rapidly to about 20 ng ml^{-1} within 5 minutes.

Peripheral Vascular Effects

Hypotension can occur after even small (10 mg) doses of IV morphine, and is primarily related to decreases in systemic vascular resistance (SVR). The most important mechanism responsible for these changes is probably histamine release. The amount of histamine release is reduced by slow administration (<10 mg min^{-1}) and histamine-induced reactions are significantly attenuated by combined H_1- and H_2-antagonist pretreatment. Morphine may have a direct action on vascular smooth muscle, independent of histamine release.[30] In the isolated hindlimbs of dogs anesthetized with halothane, high doses of alfentanil (500 μg kg^{-1}), fentanyl (50 μg kg^{-1}), and sufentanil (6 μg kg^{-1}) caused significant decreases of 48, 48, and 44 percent in peripheral vascular resistance. Neither pretreatment with naloxone nor denervation changed the responses and it was concluded that the three opioids produced vasodilatation by a direct action on vascular smooth muscle.[31] Although fentanyl-induced relaxation in the rat aorta may be mediated by α-adrenergic receptors, this effect occurs only at concentrations several hundred times higher than those encountered clinically.[32]

Cerebral vascular regulation

Endogenous opioid peptides, especially the enkephalins, are present in the cerebral perivascular nerves and in the CSF, and their concentration changes in response to stimuli that activate regulatory mechanisms of the cerebral circulation. The endogenous opioid system may thus be involved in cerebral vascular autoregulation.[33] However, under resting basal conditions, endogenous opioid peptides do not appear to participate in the regulation of cerebrovascular tone, but become active during hypoxia- or hypercapnia-induced vasodilatation.[34] The enkephalins, acting primarily on δ_2 and κ receptors, produce dilatation of pial arteries by activation of inwardly rectifying and calcium-dependent potassium ion channels and also by changes in cAMP secondary to activation of adenylyl cyclase.[35]

The effects of alfentanil, fentanyl, and sufentanil on cerebral blood flow (CBF) and intracranial pressure (ICP) have been extensively studied, with often conflicting results.[36] Increases of previously normal or only slightly elevated ICP were registered in some studies in connection with a decrease in mean arterial pressure (MAP). On the other hand, in patients with brain injury and elevated ICP opioids did not further increase ICP despite MAP decreases. The cerebral effects of opioids are dependent on several factors, e.g., age, species, ventilation, anaesthesia before and during measurements, systemic haemodynamics and underlying diseases. The probable mechanism of ICP increase during decreasing MAP is cerebral vasodilatation due to maintained autoregulation. With increasing severity of the cerebral lesion autoregulation is often disturbed. Therefore, ICP often remains unaltered despite MAP decreases. However, the resulting decrease in cerebral perfusion pressure makes such patients more susceptible to develop ischaemic neurological deficits. Induction of somatic rigidity, histamine release, cerebral vasodilatation, increased cerebral oxygen consumption, or carbon dioxide accumulation during spontaneous breathing will contribute to increases in ICP/CBF.

Naloxone as therapy for cardiovascular disturbances

In view of the mainly adverse cardiovascular effects of the endogenous opioid peptides, it is not surprising that a potential therapeutic role for the opioid antagonist, naloxone, has been sought. The use of naloxone in the treatment of shock was stimulated by the work of Holaday and Faden in the late 1970s,[37,38] and since then an extensive literature has developed documenting the protective effects of this drug in hypovolaemic and endotoxic shock in animals. These protective effects of naloxone are stereo-specific, and are manifested only by the active (-) isomer. The (+) isomer of naloxone, which lacks opioid receptor antagonistic actions, did not block ischaemia and reperfusion induced impairment of haemodynamics and ventricular function caused by occlusion of a coronary artery in dogs.[4] This indicates that the protective effects of naloxone were mediated by opioid receptors.

While the results of naloxone in animals with shock have generally been positive, the results of studies in patients have been less favourable and often inconsistent. The reason for this discrepancy between animal and human clinical studies is unclear, although it is likely that the dosage and timing of naloxone are critical factors. In almost all animal studies, naloxone has been given shortly after the induction of shock, before the animals develop multiple organ failure. In contrast, in most clinical studies, naloxone therapy has only been initiated in patients in whom shock has been established for several hours or longer, and who have not responded to more conventional treatment with fluid loading, inotropic support, etc.

In a prospective study of naloxone in patients with early hyperdynamic septic shock,[39] patients given naloxone within 7 ± 0.6 hours of developing shock showed a sustained and clinically significant haemodynamic improvement. In these patients the survival rate was 100%. In contrast patients in whom the duration of shock prior to naloxone treatment was 15 ± 4.1 hours did not respond to naloxone, and none of these patients survived. Others, however, have not found a significant effect of naloxone on survival of patients with septic shock, despite a uniform beneficial haemodynamic response to the drug.[40] The significant haemodynamic improvement in these patients was attributed to the high doses used; an initial loading bolus of 0.03 mg kg^{-1} followed by an infusion of naloxone at a rate of 0.2 mg kg^{-1} h^{-1}. High doses are thought to be necessary since naloxone has a greater affinity for the μ-opioid receptors than for δ- or κ-receptors, and many if not all of the adverse circulatory effects of the endogenous opioids are due to actions at these receptors.[3] Further, at higher doses, naloxone may have a direct positive inotropic action unrelated to antagonism of endogenous opioids.[41]

References

1. Lee AY. Endogenous opioid peptides and cardiac arrhythmias. *Int J Cardiol* 1990; 27: 145-151.
2. Wu J-P, Chen Y-T, Lee A Y-S. Opioids in myocardial ischaemia: potentiating effects of dynorphin on ischaemic arrhythmia, bradycardia and cardiogenic shock following coronary artery occlusion in the rat. *Eur Heart J* 1993; 14: 1273-1277.
3. Imai N, Kashiki M, Woolf PD, Liang C-S. Comparison of cardiovascular effects of μ- and δ-opioid receptor antagonists in dogs with congestive heart failure. *Am J Physiol* 1994; 267: H912-H917.
4. Chen YT, Lin CJ, Lee AY, Chen JS, Hwang DS. Stereospecific blocking effects of naloxone against hemodynamic compromise and ventricular dysfunction due to myocardial ischemia and reperfusion. *Int J Cardiol* 1995; 50: 125-129.
5. Slepushkin VD, Pavlenko VS, Zoloyev GK, et al. The role of enkephalins in the pathogenesis of acute myocardial infarction. *Exp Pathol* 1988; 35:129-131.
6. Zimlichman R, Gefel D, Eliahou H, et al: Expression of opioid receptors during heart ontogeny in normotensive and hypertensive rats. *Circulation* 1996; 93: 1020-1025.
7. Springhorn JP, Claycomb WC. Preproenkephalin mRNA expression in developing rat heart and in cultured ventricular cardiac muscle cells. Biochem J 1989; 258: 73-78.
8. Ouellette M, Brakier-Gingras L. Increase in the relative abundance of preproenkephalin A messenger RNA in the ventricles of cardiomyopathic hamsters. *Biochem Biophys Res Commun* 1988; 155: 449-454.
9. Rimoy GH, Wright DM, Bhaskar NK, Rubin PC. The cardiovascular and central nervous system effects in the human of U-62066E. A selective κ-opioid receptor agonist. *Eur J Clin Pharmacol* 1994; 46: 203-207.
10. Ventura C, Spurgeon H, Lakatta EG, Guarnieri C, Capogrossi MC. κ and δ opioid receptor stimulation affects cardiac myocyte function and Ca^{2+} release from an intracellular pool in myocytes and neurons. *Circ Res* 1992; 70: 66-81.
11. Wong TM, Sheng JZ, Wong NS, Tai KK. Signal transduction in the cardiac κ-receptor. *Biol Signals* 1995; 4: 174-178.
12. Xiao R-P, Pepe S, Spurgeon HA, Capogrossi MC, Lakatta EG. Opioid peptide receptor stimulation reverses β-adrenergic effects in rat heart cells. Am J Physiol 1997; 272: H797-H805.
13. Saeki T, Nishimura M, Sato N, Fujinami T, Watanabe Y. Electrophysiological demonstration and activation of μ-opioid receptors in the rabbit sinoatrial node. *J Cardiovasc Pharmacol* 1995; 26: 160-168.
14. Fontana F, Bernardi P, Pich EM, et al. Relationship between plasma atrial natriuretic factor and opioid peptide levels in healthy subjects and in patients with acute congestive heart failure. *Eur Heart J* 1993; 14: 219-225.
15. Lowe H. Zur Rolle endogener Opioide bei der Herzinsuffizienz. *Z Kardiol* 1991; 80 (Suppl 8): 47-51.
16. Llobel F, Laorden ML. Effects of morphine on atrial preparations obtained from nonfailing

and failing human hearts. *Br J Anaesth* 1996; 76: 106-110.

17. Van Vliet BJ, Ruuls SR, Drukarch B, Mulder AH, Schoffelmeer AN. Beta-adrenoceptor-sensitive adenylate cyclase is inhibited by activation of mu-opioid receptors in rat striatal neurons. *Eur J Pharmacol* 1991; 195: 295-300.

18. Flacke JW, Flacke WE, Bloor BC, et al. Histamine release by four narcotics: A double-blind study in humans. *Anesth Analg* 1987; 66: 723-730.

19. Mayer N, Zimpfer M, Raberger G, Beck A. Fentanyl inhibits the canine carotid chemoreceptor reflex. *Anesth Analg* 1989; 69: 756-762.

20. Pruett JK, Blair JR, Adams RJ. Cellular and subcellular actions of opioids in the heart. *In* Estafanous FG (ed): Opioids in Anesthesia, II. Boston, Butterworth-Heinemann, 1991, pp 61-71.

21. Blair JR, Pruett JK, Introna RP, et al. Cardiac electrophysiologic effects of fentanyl and sufentanil in canine cardiac Purkinje fibers. *Anesthesiology* 1989; 71: 565-570.

22. Pugsley MK, Saint DA, Penz MP, Walker MJ. Electrophysiological and antiarrhythmic actions of the kappa agonist PD 129290, and its R,R (+)-enantiomer, PD 129289. *Br J Pharmacol* 1993; 110: 1579-1585.

23. Saini V, Carr DB, Hagestad EL, et al. Antifibrillatory action of the narcotic agonist fentanyl. *Am Heart J* 1988; 115: 598-605.

24. Hess L, Vrana M, Vranova Z, Fejfar Z. The antifibrillatory effect of fentanyl, sufentanil and carfentanil in the acute phase of local myocardial ischaemia in the dog. *Acta Cardiol* 1989; 44: 303-311.

25. Goldberg AH, Padget CH. Comparative effects of morphine and fentanyl on isolated heart muscle. *Anesth Analg* 1969; 48: 978-982.

26. Strauer B. Contractile responses to morphine, piritramide, meperidine and fentanyl: A comparative study of effects on the isolated ventricular myocardium. *Anesthesiology* 1972; 37: 304-310.

27. Sullivan DL, Wong KC. The effects of morphine on the isolated heart during normothermia and hypothermia. *Anesthesiology* 1973; 38: 550-556.

28. Chen Zhang C, Su JY, Calkins D. Effects of alfentanil on isolated cardiac tissues of the rabbit. *Anesth Analg* 1990; 71: 268-274.

29. Kohno K, Takaki M, Ishioka K, et al. Effects of intracoronary fentanyl on left ventricular mechanoenergetics in the excised cross-circulated canine heart. *Anesthesiology* 1997; 86: 1350-1358.

30. Lowenstein E, Whiting RB, Bittar DA, Sanders CA, Powell WJ Jr. Local and neurally mediated effects of morphine on skeletal muscle vascular resistance. *J Pharmacol Exp Ther* 1972; 180: 359-367.

31. White DA, Reitan JA, Kien ND, Thorup SJ. Decrease in vascular resistance in the isolated canine hindlimb after graded doses of alfentanil, fentanyl, and sufentanil. *Anesth Analg* 1990; 71: 29-34.

32. Karasawa F, Iwanov V, Moulds RF. Effects of fentanyl on the rat aorta are mediated by alpha-adrenoceptors rather than by the endothelium. *Br J Anaesth* 1993; 71: 877-880.

33. Nagamachi K, Shitara K, Yamashita Y, et al. H Role of endogenous opioids and central opioid receptors in cerebral cortical blood flow autoregulation. *Jpn J Physiol* 1995; 45: 137-149.

34. Benyo Z, Wahl M. Opiate receptor-mediated mechanisms in the regulation of cerebral blood flow. *Cerebrovasc Brain Metab Rev* 1996; 8: 326-357.

35. Armstead WM. Role of opioids in the physiologic and pathophysiologic control of the

cerebral circulation. *Proc Soc Exp Biol Med* 1997; 214: 210-221.

36. Schregel W, Weyerer W, Cunitz G. Opioide, Hirndurchblutung und intrakranieller Druck. *Anaesthesist* 1994; 43: 421-430.

37. Holaday JW, Faden AI. Naloxone reversal of endotoxin hypotension suggests role of endorphins in shock. *Nature* 1978; 275: 450-451.

38. Faden AI, Holaday JW. Naloxone treatment of endotoxin shock: stereospecificity of physiologic and pharmacologic effects in the rat. *J Pharmacol Exp Ther* 1980; 212: 441-447.

39. Safani M, Blair J, Ross D, Waki R, Li C, Libby G. Prospective, controlled, randomized trial of naloxone infusion in early hyperdynamic septic shock. *Crit Care Med* 1989; 17: 1004-1009.

40. Hackshaw KV, Parker GA, Roberts JW. Naloxone in septic shock. *Crit Care Med* 1990; 18: 47-51.

41. Sagy M, Shavit G, Oron Y, Vidne BA, Gitter S, Sarne Y. Nonopiate effect of naloxone on cardiac muscle contractility. *J Cardiovasc Pharmacol* 1987; 9: 682-685.

Mechanisms for effects of inhalational anesthetics on control of ventilation

Denham S. Ward

General anesthesia pharmacology

Anesthesia is a clinically defined "state" that has been thought of having many quite nonspecific generalized effects besides the elimination of consciousness. When the primary anesthetic agents were inhalational agents that appeared chemically inert it made some sense to think about the "effects of anesthesia" rather than the effects of particular anesthetic drugs. Desired clinical actions from anesthetic drugs that define the clinical state of anesthesia include: "analgesia, anxiolysis, amnesia, unconsciousness, suppression of somatic motor, cardiovascular and hormonal responses to surgery and myorelaxation."[1] Interestingly, depression of respiration is not given in this definition. In fact, anesthetics have quite variable effects on ventilation, and ventilatory depression during anesthesia is relatively easily managed with endotracheal intubation and mechanical ventilation. However, depression of respiration is a common side effect of most, but not all, (*e.g.*, ketamine) anesthetics. As intravenous anesthetics have been developed, more knowledge has been obtained about specific receptor systems that can produce all or some of the characteristics of the clinical anesthetic state. Some drugs that seem to provide "complete" anesthesia do so by action at specific receptors (*e.g.*, dexmedetomidine, an agonist at α_2-receptors).[2] Different anesthetics have very different potencies for their desired effects, let alone the less desirable side effects (*e.g.*, cardiovascular and respiratory depression). For example, opioids give complete analgesia at doses that do not provide amnesia and unconsciousness while giving cardiovascular stability, but severe ventilatory depression. The benzodiazapines give anxiolysis and amnesia at doses that do not suppress somatic motor responses to pain or appreciably depress respiration.

While the potency of inhalational anesthetics have been measured by their MAC value (the minimum alveolar concentration at which 50% of the patients do not respond with a purposeful somatic motor movement when stimulated with a surgical incision), this is only one of the aspects of anesthesia. For inhalational anesthetics, the relationship between amnesia, hypnosis, somatic movement suppression, autonomic response suppression and lethal cardiovascular depression follows a predictable relationship with increasing dose. For example, at doses that suppress movement there is usually significant increases in blood pressure and heart rate following surgical stimulation. However, this relationship is not true for all anesthetic agents. The degree of respiratory stimulation with surgical stimulation in relationship to the other responses has not been well studied. The effects on respiration is, however, an important characteristic anesthetic effect. For example, opioids cause ventilation depression at far lower doses than needed to suppress somatic movement and even larger doses are required for loss of consciousness. With ketamine, analgesia is produced at lower doses than needed to cause loss of consciousness and somatic responses while ventilation is preserved (or even stimulated). The individual characteristics (both desired and side effects) of the anesthetic state are not all produced by the same relative anesthetic dose for the anesthetic agents, including the different inhalational anesthetics.

Many seemingly "inert" gases and vapors cause a loss of consciousness and the other necessary attributes for an acceptable anesthetic agent. The only commonality between many of these substances was the relationship between lipid partition coefficient and anesthetic potency that appears to be linear on a log-log scale (Meyer-Overton correlation). This relationship pointed to a lipid membrane site of action and since the agents had a variety of chemical and physical properties, indicated a nonspecific mechanism of action (*e.g.*, disruption of membrane structure). However, recent experimental evidence seems to support a more specific site of action at an intramembrane site on the $GABA_A$ receptor.[3,4] There may be similar sites on other receptors and channels.[5] For the inhalational anesthetics, the depression of respiration may be partly due to alternations of consciousness and other 'open loop' inputs to the ventilatory centers as well as depression of the chemoreflex loops through the same mechanisms that cause the anesthetic effects (*e.g.*, $GABA_A$ receptors). Of particular interest are the recent observations that the site of action that prevents movement may be in the spinal cord, while the site that causes amnesia is a central site.[6] It is becoming apparent that anesthesia, even when caused by an inhalational anesthetic, is not a nonspecific state, but rather it is the combination of very specific interactions at the cellular level.

Regulation of respiration
Because the respiratory system must perform multiple voluntary and autonomic tasks, some of which may be contradictory, the regulatory mechanisms are understandably complex. An important distinction are between open loop and closed loop inputs to the controller. The open loop inputs are the factors[7,8] (*e.g.*, body temperature, metabolic rate, pain, sleep state, and learned/conditioned responses) that effect ventilation that are themselves only weakly and indirectly effected by the level of ventilation. The closed loops inputs refer to the chemoreflex loops (*e.g.*, carotid and central chemoreceptor mediated responses to hypercapnia, hypoxia and acidemia) and the neural reflex loops (*e.g.*, vagal Hering-Baurer reflex) in which the input is strongly and directly effected by the level of ventilation.

In engineering terms a system with multiple interacting closed and open loop controls tends to be very "robust". That is, alterations in the parameters and operation of the controller may not be manifest, except by subtle changes in performance when the system is stressed, by the observable characteristics of the system. This makes it particularly problematic to discern the multiple sites of action that the general anesthetics have on the respiratory controller.

Effects of inhalational anesthetics on regulation of breathing
The primary observation is that anesthesia with inhalational agents interferes with gas exchange resulting in hypoxia and hypercapnia.[9] The degree of the depression of gas exchange is dose related, however, doses that provide adequate clinical anesthesia generally

still provide for adequate oxygenation and carbon dioxide removal. Somatic responses to painful stimulation are suppressed by a level of anesthesia that still permits an autonomic stimulation that may improve gas exchange (*e.g.,* an increase in ventilation).

Observations of patients anesthetized by inhalational agents at various doses show an increased respiratory rate with a decreased tidal volume resulting in a net decrease in ventilation; a tendency for upper airway obstruction; an apparent reduction in the ribcage contribution to ventilation; an increase in deadspace resulting in a larger increase in P_aCO_2 than would be expected from the decrease in ventilation; a reduction in the hypercapnic ventilatory response; and a marked reduction in the hypoxic ventilatory response. Some of these effects may be due to changes in the closed loop chemoreflexes, while others may reflect alterations in open loop inputs. This has made it particularly difficult to decipher the effects of low doses of inhalational anesthetics on the hypoxic ventilatory response.[10]

The use of a system of artificial perfusion of the brainstem of the cat by the group in Leiden has allowed for several interesting observations regarding possible sites of action. They found that the characteristic tachypnea of halothane occurred when halothane was introduced to the brainstem alone and started sooner than the ventilatory depression.[11] When central and peripheral CO_2 sensitivities were calculated, it was found that both were reduced when halothane was introduced either centrally or peripherally. They concluded: "... the main action of halothane is on that part of the pathways to ventilation common to both peripheral and central chemoreceptors. ... the action of halothane mainly resides in the integrating centers, the spinal motor neurons, respiratory muscles, and elastance rather in the peripheral and central chemoreceptors as such."[11] Since hypoxia has specific effects on the peripheral chemoreceptors, the Leiden investigators subsequently extended this work to hypoxia.[12] They again concluded that: "... the main depressant effect of peripheral halothane on the overall ventilatory response to CO_2 during peripheral hypoxemia is located in structures common to both the peripheral and central chemoreflex *i.e.,* the neuromechanical link between brainstem centers and respiratory movements (motorneurons, respiratory muscles, or lung elastance)."[12] Interestingly, they also noted that the combination of peripheral halothane with chloralose-urethane resulted in more reduction in ventilation than halothane both peripherally and centrally. It may be possible that a significant portion of halothane's action, in cats at least, is at the spinal cord level just as its effects on suppressing somatic movement is a spinal action.

In humans, halothane more clearly has a carotid body site of action.[13,14] It is not know what the characteristics of the human carotid body are that make them have this increased sensitivity to inhalation anesthetics. However, in humans the effects of the drive from higher centers becomes critically important,[15] but painful stimuli may have less effects.[16] This again raises the possibilities that the inhalational anesthetics may depress ventilation both with spinal cord and central (brainstem and cortical) effects. Assessing the different inhalational anesthetics at the same MAC accounts for their spinal cord potency, but they may have different central actions which could account for their different effects on the hypoxic ventilatory response.[16]

Conclusion

Much is being learned about both specific sites of action (both for particular organs and at subcellular sites) of the inhalational anesthetics and that some of these sites may correlate with the components of the anesthetic state. In addition, there is exciting new information available regarding specific sites of the action of inhalational anesthetics on specific receptor molecules. This work will enable the respiratory effects of the inhalational anesthetics to be studied in much more detail.

References

1.   Kissin I. A concept for assessing interactions of general anaesthetics. *Anesth Analg* 85: 204-210, 1997.
2.   Ward DS, Temp JA. Neuropharmacology of the control of ventilation. In: *Anesthesia: Biologic Foundations*, edited by Biebuyck J, Lynch C, Maze M, et al. Philadelphia: Lippincott-Raven, 1997, p. 1367-1394.
3.   Mihic SJ, Ye Q, Wick MJ, et al. Sites of alcohol and volatile anesthetic action on $GABA_A$ and glycine receptors. *Br J Anaesth* 71: 29-38, 1997.
4.   Tanelian DL, Kosek P, Mody I, et al. The role of the $GABA_A$ receptor/chloride channel complex in anesthesia. *Anesthesiology* 78: 757-776, 1993.
5.   Urban BW. Differential effects of gaseous and volatile anaesthetics on sodium and potassium channels. *Br. J. Anaesth* 71: 29-38, 1993.
6.   Eger EI, Koblin DD, Harris RA, et al. Hypothesis: Inhaled anesthetics produce immobility and amnesia by different mechanisms at different sites. *Anesth Analg* 84: 915-918, 1997.
7.   Shea SA. Behavioral and arousal-related influences on breathing in humans. *Exp Physiol* 81: 1-26, 1996.
8.   Douglas NJ, White DP, Weil JV, et al. Hypoxic ventilatory response decreases during sleep in normal man. *Am. Rev Respir Dis* 125: 286-289, 1982.
9.   Nunn JF. Effects of anaesthesia on respiration. *Br J Anaesth* 65: 54-62, 1990.
10.   Ward DS. Inhalational anesthetics and control of breathing during hypoxia. *Anesth Clin North Am* 1998.(In Press).
11.   Berkenbosch A, DeGoede J, Olievier CN, et al. Sites of action of halothane on respiratory pattern and ventilatory response to CO_2 in cats. *Anesthesiology* 57: 389-398, 1982.
12.   van Dissel JT, Berkenbosch A, Olievier CN, et al. Effects of halothane on the ventilatory response to hypoxia and hpercapnia in cats.. *Anesthesiology* 62: 448-456, 1985.
13.   Knill RL Gelb AW. Ventilatory responses to hypoxia and hypercapnia during halothane sedation and anesthesia in man. *Anesthesiology* 49: 244-251, 1978.
14.   Dahan A, van den Elsen MJLJ, Berkenbosch A, et al. Effects of subanesthetic halothane on the ventilatory responses to hypercapnia and acute hypoxia in healthy volunteers. *Anesthesiology* 80: 727-738, 1994.
15.   van den Elsen MJLJ, Dahan A, Berkenbosch A, et al. Does subanesthetic isoflurane affect the ventilatory response to acute isocapnic hypoxia in healthy volunteers?. *Anesthesiology* 81: 860-867, 1994.
16.   Sarton E, Dahan A, Teppema L, et al. Acute pain and central nervous system arousal do not restore impaired hypoxic ventilatory response during sevoflurane sedation. *Anesthesiology* 85: 295-303, 1996.

Opioid-induced analgesia and respiratory depression: Sex differences

Benjamin Kest, Elise Sarton, Jeffrey S. Mogil, and Albert Dahan

Introduction

Exogenous opioids such as morphine exert powerful physiological effects, including analgesia and respiratory depression. These effects exhibit marked inter-individual differences, however. In addition to the well-documented effects of age/development and genetic background, the contribution of sex and hormonal status as a factor in opioid potency is becoming increasingly appreciated. Progress in this area has been slow, perhaps since most studies on the analgesic and respiratory effects of opioids utilize male subjects to avoid the need to control for estrous/menstrual status. Additionally, sex differences in opioid analgesia have been reported by some to be either negligible or absent. This may reflect differences in the methodology-species, strain and age of the animals, particular nociceptive assay employed and its parameters–employed by each laboratory. Nonetheless, findings from an increasing number of studies directly examining the issue of sex and hormonal status in the potency of opioids demonstrate that sex and hormonal factors need to be considered if opioid drugs are to be used in the most efficacious manner possible.

Analgesia

Animal Studies. The systemic administration of morphine produces greater peak or total analgesia in male relative to female rats[2, 14, 23] and mice,[11, 27, 28, 29] although non-significant differences have also been reported in rats.[1, 23, 26] The enhanced sensitivity of males to morphine analgesia has been documented across several pain tests, including those assessing thermal and somatic (hot-plate[14, 27, 35] and tail-flick/withdrawal tests[11, 14, 23, 31]) chemical and visceral (abdominal writhing following acetic acid[14] or hypertonic saline,[2] and electric shock (jump test[31]) nociception. Sex differences in opioid analgesia may be mediated by enhanced central nervous system (CNS) sensitivity to opioids since males display lower half-maximal analgesia (ED_{50}) values than females following central administration of morphine and/or the enkephalin-derived opioid DAMGO ([D-Ala^2, N-Me-Phe^4, Gly-ol^5]-enkephalin) via the intracerebroventricular (icv) route in rats[31, 32] and mice.[33, 34] Although DAMGO and morphine act primarily at the μ-opioid receptor type, the effect of sex on μ-opioid analgesia remains equivocal since Bartok and Craft[4] observed no differences between males and female rats following fentanyl or buprenorphine on either the hot-plate or tail-withdrawal assay. Furthermore, although male rats displayed significantly greater DAMGO analgesic magnitude on the tail-flick test relative to females,[32] regression analysis failed to reveal significant potency differences related to sex, and sex differences were not observed on the jump test. Thus, sex differences in μ-opioid analgesia may depend on route of administration, nociceptive assay employed, and method of quantifying analgesia.

The magnitude and direction of sex differences in morphine analgesia appears to vary with other organismic factors, such as genotype. For example, male Sprague-Dawley and Wistar-Furth rats both displayed greater morphine analgesia than females following systemic administration, and sex-related potency differences varied in magnitude between these strains.[26] In a comparison of inbred male and female mice, no significant sex differences in analgesia were observed in the majority of 11 strains examined following central administration of morphine.[34] However, morphine analgesia was significantly greater in males of three strains, and significantly greater in females of one strain. In a study examining central DAMGO analgesia in mice bi-directionally selected from Swiss-Webster stock for high (HA) and low (LA) stress-induced analgesia, HA but not LA males displayed greater analgesic potency than their female counterparts.[33] Age has also been shown to interact with sex in the modulation of morphine analgesia. Whereas there is an age-related enhancement of peak and total (area under the curve) morphine analgesia in male rats, female rats display an age-related decline, although at a low dose females may actually show an enhanced response.[23] Finally, sex differences are subject to circadian fluctuation in mice, being maximal during the dark period, with nocturnal opioid sensitivity markedly greater in males.[27]

Sex differences in the analgesic effects of opioids acting at the κ- and δ-opioid receptor types have also been reported. Similar to μ-opioid receptor-mediated analgesia, sex differences may be assay-, dose-, and/or time-dependent. Following administration of the κ-receptor-selective opioid, U69,593, in rats, a significant sex by time interaction was noted on the tail-withdrawal test (peak effect: females 5-15 min, males 30 min post-injection), but no sex differences were observed on the hot-plate test.[4] In the same study, the κ-agonist bremazocine produced somewhat *greater* analgesia in females compared to males at some dose and time points on both assays. Sex differences in κ-opioid analgesia is also observed in mice, with males displaying greater analgesia than females on the hot-plate following the κ-selective opioid, U-50,488H.[27] Using the enkephalin-derived opioid, DSLET, Kepler et al.[32] reported no effect of sex on δ-opioid analgesia on the tail-flick or hot-plate test. However, recent work using more selective δ-opioids reveal a different pattern. Both DPDPE and deltorphin, selective δ_1- and δ_2-opioid receptor agonists, respectively, produced significant sex by dose interactions on the hot-plate but not tail-flick test, with significantly less analgesia in female relative to male rats.[4] Additionally, peak DPDPE analgesia also differed between males (15-30 min post-injection) and females (5 min post-injection).

The mechanism(s) underlying sex differences in opioid analgesia remains elusive. The greater availability of morphine to the brain of male mice relative to females following systemic injections suggests that sex differences may be simply related to differences in opioid pharmacokinetics.[11] However, no differences in morphine serum levels are observed between sex in rats assayed at post-injection latencies corresponding to peak morphine analgesic effect.[14] Pharmacokinetic explanations of sex differences in opioid analgesia are further discounted given the greater analgesia observed in male mice[33, 34] and rats [31, 32] even following icv opioid administration. Sex differences in opioid analgesia are also not likely related to differences in supraspinal opioid receptor density since no differences in brain μ-

and δ-opioid receptor populations are observed between male and female rats.[31] In mice, both increased levels in males[37] and no differences[11] in opioid binding between sexes have been reported. Finally, the relationship between opioid receptor density and sex differences in analgesia is questioned by the report that male mice undergo greater up-regulation of morphine analgesia than females following chronic opioid antagonist treatment with naltrexone despite no effect of sex on the degree of opioid receptor up-regulation.[11] Sex differences in opioid analgesia may also result from differences in the endogenous neurochemical systems that influence morphine analgesia. For example, there is evidence indicating that N-methyl-D-aspartate (NMDA)-sensitive excitatory amino acid receptors mediate morphine analgesia in mice[35] and rats,[24] but selective NMDA receptor blockade significantly reduces morphine analgesia in male mice only.[35] The endogenous opioid peptides leu- and met-enkephalin can also affect morphine potency,[47] and sex differences in their immunoreactive density has been demonstrated in the rat.[45,48] Male and female mice may also differ in the activity of the proteolytic enzymes that limit endogenous opioid peptide activity, since the antinociceptive effects of enkephalinase inhibition is more pronounced in males.[30] Sex differences in the anti-opioid effects of the endogenous peptides Tyr-MIF-1 and neuropeptide FF on morphine analgesia in mice have also been noted.[28,29]

Not surprisingly, many investigators have attempted to relate sex differences in opioid analgesia with the activity of gonadal hormones. For example, simulating pregnancy concentrations of 17-*B* estradiol and progesterone in non-pregnant rats increased responsiveness to spinally administered U-50,488H.[17] Intact rats are also more sensitive to the analgesic effects of systemic morphine on the mornings of diestrous[3] and proestrous,[3,5] though in mice there does not appear to be variation in opioid sensitivity across the estrous cycle.[39] Estrous effects on central morphine analgesia in rats are also observed, with significantly greater analgesic magnitude occurring during proestrous and estrous, but estrous phase in general failed to alter the dose-response function.[32] Studies with gonadectomized subjects are less clear. Whereas increased morphine analgesia following systemic administration is observed in ovariectomized females relative to sham-operated controls on the hot-plate,[1] there was no significant effect in a visceral nociceptive assay.[2] On this basis it might be argued that gonadal hormones may have differential effects on different nociceptive modalities. However, although adult ovariectomy has been reported to reduce the magnitude but not potency of morphine analgesia on the tail-flick test in rats following central[31] and systemic[3] administration, morphine analgesia following systemic administration has also been reported to be increased[26] or not changed.[14] Thus, conflicting results are observed even when nociceptive assay is held constant. Exposure to estradiol or progesterone replacement therapy in ovariectomized rats caused reductions in morphine analgesia on the hot-plate test, although the effect of the lower progesterone dose varied with time of treatment.[42] The effect of gonadectomy on morphine analgesia in male rats and mice are also equivocal. There are reports of both reduced[12] and unaltered[14,26] systemic morphine analgesia for rats on the tail-flick test following castration. Again, the effects of castration may be nociceptive modality-specific since increased morphine analgesia on the hot-plate is also observed.[1] Like female rats, central morphine analgesia on the tail-flick and jump tests are reduced in magnitude but not potency in male rats following gonadectomy.[31]

In male mice, morphine analgesia is increased on the hot-plate test and against abdominal writhing induced by acetic acid,[1] but decreased on the tail-flick test,[11] following castration. Testosterone was effective in reversing the attenuated morphine sensitivity of the castrated rat.[12] In fact, whereas estradiol 17-*B* and progesterone had no significant effect on morphine potency in intact male rats, testosterone produced biphasic effects, first potentiating (30 min) then attenuating (4 h) systemic morphine analgesia.[12] Testosterone, but not estradiol 17-*B* or progesterone alone or in combination, also restored morphine potency in ovariectomized rats and rats in post-partum, when normal ovarian activity is halted.[3] These findings suggest that testosterone regulates morphine sensitivity in female rats. However, the progesterone metabolite 17-*α*-hydroxyprogesterone had no effect on morphine analgesia per se, but antagonized the effect of testosterone in restoring morphine sensitivity in ovariectomized rats,[3] suggesting an interaction between ovarian steroids in modulating morphine potency. Finally, ovariectomy eliminated the age-related attenuation (see above) in the potency and magnitude of morphine analgesia relative to intact females, but had only marginal effects on the increased morphine analgesia observed in aged males.[23] It should be noted however, that sex steroids can exert widespread short- and long-term effects on cellular physiology and organization, and significant variability exists between studies with regards to the age of the animals at the time of, and the latencies between, ovariectomy, hormone replacement therapy, and nociceptive testing. Thus, the lack of uniform methodology may again contribute to the apparent confusion in the literature.

Apparent inconsistencies notwithstanding, the mechanism by which gonadal hormonal milieu may modulate opioid analgesia remains unknown. For example, there are conflicting reports regarding the effect of castration on opioid receptor integrity. Whereas increased receptor density has been reported for rats,[22] other groups report no changes in opioid receptor density or affinity in rats and mice.[11, 13, 18] In female rats, ovarian steroid treatment and ovariectomy alters brain opioid binding sites.[41,50] This regulation may occur at the level of the gene as progesterone increases levels of μ-opioid receptor mRNA in hypothalamic regions of ovariectomized, estradiol-treated rats.[41] However, as noted above, it is unlikely that sex differences in opioid receptor binding in intact mice or rats is a viable explanation for sex differences in analgesia. Kepler et al.[31] have suggested that gonadal hormones may regulate opioid receptor function via interactions between co-localized central opioid and gonadal steroid receptors in areas relevant to opioid analgesia like the mesencephalic central gray and amygdala. Additional sites of possible interaction suggested by these authors[31] include the central steroid receptors localized in areas of the hypothalamus, where the density of immunoreactive serotonin and the opioid peptides leu- and met-enkephalin display sexual dimorphism.[44,45,48] These transmitters have been shown to modulate morphine analgesia.[19,43,47] The nature of these interactions, if they indeed exist, and their relevance to opioid analgesia are currently unknown.

Human Studies. That patient variables such as sex need to be considered in pain treatment protocols gains support from the finding that, for a given opioid treatment protocol for metastatic cancer, only females reported inadequate pain relief.[15] Still, sex-differences in opioid analgesia in humans has been greatly understudied. Additionally, comparisons across studies are difficult since patients typically vary widely in many variables that can affect analgesic efficacy, including patient age,[10, 15] personality,[9] and type, duration and progression of the disease/pain.[8] Indeed, sex differences in pain perception per se has been the subject of recent review.[6] A further problem inherent in the study of opioid analgesia in human subjects is that the controlled administration of opioids, and the examination of their effects on objective nociceptive assays, is generally not practical. Studies are thus typically comprised of post-hoc comparisons of patient requests for analgesics. For example, following hip replacement surgery, women requested the opioid analgesic buprenorphine less often than men.[36] More female than male cancer patients found adequate pain relief from low doses of diamorphine, although more women were also prescribed an anxiolytic.[46] However, where the variability in the analgesic effect of graded doses of intramuscular morphine to control cancer pain was studied, no differences were attributable to sex of the patient.[25] Furthermore, no sex differences in morphine analgesia was observed in patients undergoing standardized surgery for the removal of third molar teeth.[21] In two separate studies, however, analgesia produced by the κ-opioids pentazocine, nalbuphine, and butorphanol for molar extraction was greater in females.[20,21] A potential confound in human studies is the influence of social sex role expectancies in pain perception and/ on pain reporting,[8] resulting in a differential reluctance or tendency between men and women in requesting pain relief. However, in a study of patient-controlled morphine analgesia, where social stigma attached to narcotic request is presumably minimized, differing results are obtained. Whereas there was no effect of sex on narcotic usage for pain following iliac crest bone grafting of alveolar clefts,[16] men required significantly more morphine following abdominal surgery.[10] In a recent experimental study in which cutaneous nociceptors were activated by transcutaneous electrical stimulation on the skin overlying the tibial bone, a significant reduction of the numerical rating score for pain after intravenous morphine occurred in men but not in women (A. Dahan, personal communication).

Collectively, these studies demonstrate that opioid analgesia sex differences in humans, like in animals, may depend on the interaction of several variables, including age, type of pain, and opioid pharmacodynamics.

Respiration

Among the many side effect of opioids, especially of μ-opioid receptor agonists, respiratory depression is most serious. Surprisingly, no studies in animals and only few studies in humans considered the influence of sex on opioid-induced respiratory depression. In a study on adverse respiratory events during conscious sedation in a pediatric population the combined administration of the μ-agonist fentanyl and the benzodiazepine midazolam caused respiratory depression in 11% of patients.[51] Significantly more (and more serious) respiratory events occurred in female patients (odds ratio = 2.2).

Recently, Dahan and coworkers showed qualitative and quantitative sex-related differences in morphine-induced respiratory depression in young, healthy adults.[52] Morphine caused more severe depression of ventilatory responses to hypoxia and hypercapnia in women compared to men. In women, the depression of ventilatory responses by morphine was not related to the phase of the menstrual cycle. In both sexes, morphine-induced changes were unrelated to weight, height, fat mass and sex hormone concentrations.

The scarce data on sex differences in opioid-induced alterations of ventilatory control make it difficult to hypothesize on possible mechanisms. The data of Dahan and coworkers[52] point towards the peripheral chemoreflex loop as site for sex differences. Since the carotid bodies posses μ-opioid receptors, it may well be that the sex differences observed in the above mentioned studies[51, 52] originate at peripheral chemoreceptors themselves.

Conclusions

It is clear that under certain conditions, opioids can exert differential effects in males and females. However, the direction and magnitude of these differences seems dependent on many interacting variables. How can the relative contribution of these variables be sorted out? Which are the most relevant for differences in sensitivity between sex? Using a quantitative trait loci (QTL) mapping strategy, Mogil and colleagues[37] have recently identified a chromosomal region associated with the non-opioid stress-induced analgesic response in females only. This region accounts for 18-26% of the overall trait variance in this sex. We are currently in the process of the QTL mapping of morphine analgesia in mice of both sexes in the hope of identifying confirmatory and/or heuristic information regarding the physiological mechanisms underlying sex differences.

Evidently, when future studies indicate that sex is an important factor in opioid-induced analgesia in humans, we will have to take this into account when administrating opioids for pain relief and apply separate analgesic regimens for men and women directed at the ideal combination of optimal pain relief with minimal respiratory depression.

References

1. Ali B, Sharif S, Elkadi A: Sex differences and the effect of gonadectomy on morphine-induced antinociception and dependence in rats and mice. *Clin Exp Pharmacol Physiol* 1995; 22: 342-4
2. Baamonde AI, Hidalgo A, Adrés-Trelles F: Sex-related differences in the effects of morphine and stress on visceral pain. *Neuropharmacol* 1989; 28: 967-70
3. Banarjee P, Chatterjee TK, Ghosh JJ: Ovarian steroids and modulation of morphine-induced analgesia and catalepsy in female rats. *Eur J Pharmacol* 1983; 96: 291-4
4. Bartok RE, Craft RM: Sex differences in opioid antinociception. *J Pharmacol Exp Ther* 1997; 282: 769-78
5. Berglund LA, Simpkins JW: Alterations in brain opiate receptor mechanisms on proestrous afternoon. *Neuroendocrin* 1988; 48: 394-400
6. Berkely KJ: Sex differences in pain. *Behav Brain Sci* 1997; 20: 371-80
7. Bodnar RJ, Romeo M-T, Kramer E: Organismic variables and pain inhibition: roles of gender and aging. *Brain Res Bull* 1988; 21: 947-53
8. Bond MR, Pilowsky I: Subjective assessment of pain and its relationship to the administration of analgesics in patients with advanced cancer. *J Psychosom Res* 1966; 10: 203-8
9. Boyle P, Parbrook GD: The interrelation of personality on post-operative factors. *Br J Anaesth* 1977; 49: 259-64
10. Burns JW, Hodsman NBA, McLIntock TTC, Gillies GWA, Kenny GNC, McArdle CS: The influence of patient characteristic on the requirements for postoperative analgesia. *Anaes* 1989; 44: 2-6
11. Candido J, Lufty K, Billings B, Sierra V, Duttaroy A, Inturrisi CE, Yoburn BC: Effect of

adrenal and sex hormones on opioid analgesia and opioid receptor regulation. *Pharmacol Biochem Behav* 1992; 42: 685-92

12. Chatterjee TK, Das S, Banarjee P, Ghosh JJ: Possible physiological role of adrenal and gonadal steroids in morphine analgesia. *Eur J Pharmacol* 1982; 77: 119-23

13. Cicero TJ, Newman KS, Meyer ER: testosterone does not influence opiate binding sites in the male rat brain. *Life Sci* 1983; 33: 1231-9

14. Cicero TJ, Nock B, Meyer ER: Gender-related differences in the antinociceptive properties of morphine. *J Pharmacol Exp Ther* 1996; 279: 763-73

15. Cleeland CS, Gonin R, Hatfield AK, Edmonson JH, Blum RH, Stewart JA, Pandya KJ: Pain and its treatment in outpatients with metastatic cancer. *New Eng J Med* 1998; 330: 592-6

16. Dawson KH, Egbert MA, Myall RW: Pain following iliac crest bone grafting of alveolar clefts. *J Pharmacol Exp Ther* 1996; 24: 151-4

17. Dason-Basoa M, Gintzler AR: Estrogen and progesterone activate spnial kappa-opiate receptor analgesic mechanisms. *Pain* 1996; 64: 169-77

18. Diez JA, Roberts JL: Evidence contradicting the notion that gonadal hormones regulate brain opiate receptors. *Biochem Biophys Res Comm* 1982; 108: 1313-9

19. Fields HL, Heinricher MM, Mason P: Neurotransmitters in nociceptive modulatory circuits. *Annu Rev Neurosci* 1991; 14: 219-45

20. Gear RW, Miakowski C, Gordon NC, Paul SM, Heller PH, Levine JD: Kappa-opioids produce significantly greater analgesia in women than in men. *Nature Med* 1995; 11: 1248-50

21. Gordon NC, Gear RW, Heller PH, Paul S, Miakowski C, Levine JD. Enhancement of morphine analgesia by $GABA_B$ agonist baclofen. *Neurosci* 1995; 69: 345-9

22. Hahn EF, Fishman J: Castration affects male rat brain opiate receptor content. *Neuroendocrin* 1985; 41: 60-3

23. Islam AK, Cooper ML, Bodnar RJ: Interactions among aging, gender and gonadectomy affects upon morphine antinociception in rats. *Physiol Behav* 1993; 54: 43-54

24. Jacquet YF: The NMDA receptor: central role in pain inhibition in rat periaqueductal gray. *Eut J Pharmacol* 1988; 154: 271-6

25. Kaiko RF, Wallenstein SL, Rogers AG, Houde RW: Sources of variation in analgesic responses in cancer patients with chronic pain receiving morphine. *Pain* 1983; 15: 191-200

26. Kasson BG, George R: Endocrine influences on the actions of morphine . IV. Effects of sex and strain. *Life Sci* 1984; 34: 1627-34

27. Kavaliers M, Innes DGL: Sex and day-night differences in opiate-induced responses of insular wild deer mice, *peromyscus maniculatus triangularis. Pharmacol Biochem Behav* 1987; 27: 477-82

28. Kavaliers M, Innes DGL: Sex differences in the effects of Tyr-MIF-1 on morphine- and stress-induced analgesia. *Peptides* 1992; 13: 1295-7

29. Kavaliers M, Innes DGL: Sex differences in the effects of neuropeptide FF and IgG from neuropeptide FF on morphine- and stress-induced analgesia. *Peptides* 1992; 13: 603-7

30. Kavaliers M, Innes DGL: Sex differences in the antinociceptive effects of the enkephalinase inhibitor SCH 34826. *Pharmacol Biochem Behav* 1993; 46: 777-80

31. Kepler KL, Kest B, Kiefel JM, Cooper ML, Bodnar RJ: Roles of gender, gonadectomy and estrous phase in the analgesic effects of intracerebroventricular morphine in rats. *Pharmacol Biochem Behav* 1989; 34: 119-27

32. Kepler KL, Standifer KM, Paul D, Kest B, Pasternak GW, Bodnar RJ: Gender effects and central opioid analgesia. *Pain* 1991; 45: 87-94

33. Kest B, Brodsky M, Sadowski B, Mogil JS, Inturrisi CE: Mu opioid receptor (MOR-1) mRNA

levels are altered in mice with differential analgesic sensitivity to the mu opioid DAMGO. *Analgesia* 1995; 1: 498-501

34. Kest B, Wilson SG, Mogil JS: Genetic mediation of supraspinal morphine analgesia: strain and sex differences. 1998; in preparation

35. Lipa SM. Kavaliers M: Sex differences in the inhibitory effects of the NMDA antagonist MK-801 on morphine and stress-induced analgesia. *Brain Res Bull* 1990; 24: 627-30

36. McQuay HJ, Bullingham RES, Paterson GMC, Moore RA: Clinical effects of buprenorphine during and after operation. *Br J Anaesth* 1980; 52: 1013-9

37. Mogil JS, Marek P, O'Toole LA, Helms ML, Sadowski B, Liebeskind JC, Belknap JK: Mu-opiate receptor binding is upregulated in mice selectively bred for high stress-induced analgesia. *Brain Res* 1994; 853: 16-22

38. Mogil JS, Richards SP, O'Toole LA, Helms ML, Mitchell SR, Kest B, Belknap JK: Identification of a sex-specific quantitative trait locus mediating nonopioid stress-induced analgesia in female mice. *J Neurosci* 1997; 20: 7995-8002

39. Moskowitz AS, Terman GW, Carter KR, Morgan MJ, Liebeskind JC: Analgesic, locomotor and lethal effects of morphine in the mouse: strain comparisons. *Brain Res* 1985; 361: 46-51

40. Parsons CG, Czlonkowski A, Stein C, Herz A: Peripheral opioid receptors mediating antinociception in inflammation: activation by endogenous opioids and the role of the pituitary-adrenal axis. *Pain* 1990; 41: 81-93

41. Petersen SL, LaFlamme KD: Progesterone increases levels of μ-opioid receptor mRNA in the preoptic area and arcuate nucleus of ovariectomized, estradiol-treated female rats. *Mol Brain Res* 1997; 52: 32-7

42. Ratka A, Simpkins JW: Effects of estradiol and progesterone on the sensitivity to pain on morphine-induced antinociception in female rats. *Horm Behav* 1991; 25: 217-28

43. Schul R, Frenk H: The role of serotonin in analgesia elicited by morphine in the periaqueductal gray matter (PAG). *Brain Res* 1991; 553: 353-7

44. Simerly RB, Swanson L, Gorski RA: Demonstration of a sexual dimorphism in the distribution of serotonin-immunoreactive fibers in the medial preoptic nucleus of the rat. *J Comp Neurol* 1984; 225: 151-66

45. Simerly RB, McCall LD, Watson SJ: Distribution of opioid peptides in the pre-optic region: immunohistochemical evidence for a steroid-sensitive enkephalin sexual dimorphism. *J Comp Neurol* 1988; 276: 442-59

46. Twycross RG: Choice of strong analgesic in terminal cancer: diamorphine or morphine? *Pain* 1977; 3: 93-104

47. Vaught JL, Takemori AE: Differential effects of leucine and methionine enkephalin on morphine-induced analgesia, acute tolerance and dependence. *J Pharmacol Exp Ther* 1979; 208: 86-90

48. Watson RE, Hoffmann GE, Wiegand SJ: Sexually dimorphic opioid distribution in the preoptic area: manipulation by gonadal steroids. *Brain Res* 1986; 398: 157-63

49. Weiland NG, Wise PM: Estrogen and progesterone regulate opiate receptor densities in multiple brain regions. *Endocrin* 1990; 126: 804-8

50. Wilkinson M, Brawer JR, Wilkinson DA: Gonadal steroid-induced modification of opiate binding sites in anterior hypothalamus of female rats. *Biol Reprod* 1985; 32: 501-6

51. Graff KJ, Kennedy RM, Jaffe DM: Conscious sedation for pediatric orthopedic emergencies. *Ped Emer Care* 1996; 12: 31-5

52. Dahan A, Sarton E, Teppema L, Olievier C: Sex-related differences in the influence of morphine on ventilatory control in humans. *Anesthesiology* 1998; 88: 903-913

Separate effects of respiratory stimuli and depressants on abdominal muscle action

G. B. Drummond

Introduction and review

When considering the factors that control respiration, most studies use either ventilation or phrenic nerve output as a summary measure of ventilatory output. However, in recent years it has become clear that the respiratory muscle control may not be uniform, and that different respiratory stimuli may change the respiratory muscle drive in different ways. For example, the hypoglossal nerve and phrenic nerve have different responses to changes in peripheral and central stimuli. Carotid sinus nerve section decreases hypoglossal activity more than phrenic, and local medullary cooling to reduce central chemoreceptor activity has the opposite effect.[1] Since these nerves control muscles that play different parts in the respiratory process, it is likely that their pattern of activation would be different, but this does not account for differences in response to stimuli.

The motor pathways to the diaphragm and the abdominal muscles pass via different parts of the spinal cord. Bilateral lesions in the lateral part of the upper cervical cord reduce diaphragm activity, whereas abdominal muscle action is maintained. Similarly the pathways that control ventilatory functions of the abdominal muscles are separate from those that control other functions of the abdominal muscles, such as cough and defaecation.[2] Clearly the respiratory muscles can be activated independently, and different stimuli do not necessarily cause the same degree of activation of these muscles. The individual abdominal muscles are not activated synchronously during breathing. The transversus abdominis is the most readily activated.[3]

The abdomen is normally active during quiet breathing, at least in the upright position[4] and in some subjects this activity is phasic.[5] Abdominal muscle action is often a prominent feature of respiratory stimulation, either when respiratory effort induced voluntarily,[6] or during stimulation by hypercapnia or hypoxia,[7] in exercise[2] or by positive airway pressure.[8] The responses of the inspiratory and expiratory muscles to hypoxia and hypercapnia appear to differ.[7, 9-13]

Early studies of breathing during carbon dioxide stimulation and exercise showed that in some subjects the abdominal muscles reduce abdominal and lung volume, and reciprocally increase the dimensions of the ribcage.[14,15] Positive airway pressure has a dose dependent effect in increasing ventilation, abdominal muscle activity and the electrical activation of the diaphragm.[16] Sleep reduces the response to positive airway pressure, and the response to positive airway pressure is more pronounced when ventilation is increased.[8]

Restriction of abdominal movement in the upright subject increases the pressure that can be generated by the diaphragm during rapid activation.[17] When abdominal impedance is increased, the velocity of contraction of the diaphragm is reduced.[18]

During exercise in the upright position, the end-expiratory lung volume is reduced below FRC both during exercise [19] and also during inspiratory muscle loading.[20] The decrease is greater with more loading, and can reduce the inspiratory muscle work by up to 20%.[21] When the abdominal muscles are active at the end of expiration, their effects can resemble the effects of incomplete expiration.[22] After maximal isocapnic ventilation for two minutes, abdominal muscle fatigue can occur, as shown by a decrease in the rate of decay of abdominal pressure after a short voluntary activation.[23] Slowing of the maximum relaxation rate of muscle is a feature of fatigue.[24]

The mechanical effects of abdominal muscle action
The effects of diaphragm contraction on the relative pressure changes in pleural and abdominal pressure depends on the relative compliances of the chest wall and lung, thus:

$$\Delta P_{el}/\Delta P_{ab} = C_w/C_l$$

If the volume of the abdominal compartment changes, then there is no longer a single relationship between the volume of the ribcage and volume of the lung, and the relationship between abdominal and transpulmonary pressures also alters, so that the equation above is altered.[25] Separation of these influences may be difficult if there are rapid changes in abdominal volume and compliance, for example at the onset of inspiration. Consequently the abdominal muscles may contribute some of the force associated with tidal breathing. The exact contribution from the abdominal muscles depends on the mechanical interaction with the ribcage. Direct traction of the muscles on the ribcage has an expiratory effect, whereas increases in abdominal pressure act through the zone of apposition of the diaphragm to the lower ribcage to exert a predominantly inspiratory force. These effects may vary between species, because of differences in the shape of the ribcage.[26] Abdominal muscle activation can contribute directly to ventilation, as can be seen by the onset of inspiratory flow before the diaphragm becomes active.[27]

Abdominal muscle action can contribute to ventilation considerably in some species. For example, in the horse, expiration is clearly biphasic, with active expiration in the second phase, generated by abdominal muscle action,followed by a phase of passive inspiration when these muscles relax. This pattern of activity reduces elastic work and may contribute to up to 50% of ventilation at rest.[28]

In the dog, transversus abdominis is the predominant expiratory abdominal muscle [29] and during barbiturate anaesthesia it is activated by expiratory threshold loads, chemical stimulation by CO_2, and placing the dog in the upright position. In conscious dogs, exercise is associated with an increase in tonic abdominal expiratory activity [30] whereas hypercapnia causes an increase in phasic, expiratory activity only.[31] However hypercapnia does not lead to increased lengthening of the abdominal muscles at end-inspiration, whereas these muscles are considerably stretched during passive lung inflation. This suggests that when the muscles are stimulated with hypercapnia there may be a tonic component to the increased abdominal activity.[32] In dogs anaesthetized with pentobarbital, abdominal muscle activity increased progressively with time despite stable levels of anaesthesia and arterial PCO_2. Rib cage motion increased and the tidal volume increased, whereas the inspiratory muscle activity remained constant.[33]

Cervical vagotomy markedly attenuates resting activity and the responses to carbon dioxide and hypoxia. In many other experimental circumstances, abdominal muscle action is reduced or abolished by vagotomy,[34-40] but not all studies have found vagal activity to be necessary for abdominal muscle action.[10,12]

In the newborn pig, vagal section has little effect on the responses of the abdominal muscle to hypercapnia.[41] In an elegant study in awake lambs, the response of the intercostal muscles was proportionally more than the diaphragm when the stimulation included hypercapnia.[42]

Two types of expiratory muscle

Although both the triangularis sterni and the abdominal muscles are expiratory in effect, they respond in different ways to stimuli. Thus, hypercapnia is a more potent stimulus to the abdominal muscles, a vagal stimulus such as end-inspiratory occlusion stimulates triangularis sterni but has no effect on the abdomen, and oesophageal distension stimulates the triangularis sterni but inhibits the abdomen.[43] Localised cooling of the ventrolateral medulla in supine dogs anaesthetised with pentobarbitone can also result in different responses of the trianularis sterni and the abdominal expiratory muscles. This cooling has an effect similar to a loss of central chemoreceptor drive and causes the onset of tonic activity in the traingularis sterni and suppression of abdominal muscle activity.[44]

Effects of hypoxia

Progressive hypoxia has a virtually parallel stimulatory effect on the costal, crural diaphragm and the parasternal intercostals.[45] Carotid body activation also increases abdominal muscle activity[46] and abdominal muscle activation by peripheral hypoxia is prevented by vagotomy.[47] In contrast to the effects of peripheral hypoxia, central hypoxia reduces activation of both inspiratory and expiratory muscles.[48]

In tissue slice preparations, most rat brain cells are are depressed by hypoxia. In contrast, ventrolateral medullary neurones associated with thoracic motoneurones are stimulated by hypoxia, and these responses are not reduced after synaptic blockade with low Ca^{++} and low Mg^{++} perfusate, suggesting that this effect is the result of direct stimulation.[49]

Hypercapnia

Hypercapnia appears to have a different effect on different types of central neurones. In the cat, CO_2 causes greater responses in inspiratory than in expiratory bulbospinal neurones.[9] In awake dogs, although carotid body stimulation increases both inspiratory and expiratory muscle action, abdominal activation appears to be dependent on the level of carbon dioxide: hypocapnia suppressed mild stimulation but was not sufficient to augment more extreme hyperpnoea.[50]

Hypercapnia appears to be a more potent stimulus than hypoxia to the activation of the abdomen both during consciousness[51] and anaesthesia[12] but another study found no difference.[52] The responses to hypercapnia are generally associated with greater tidal volumes.[53] The abdominal muscles appear to be reflexly activated by increased tidal volume. In conscious dogs where abdominal muscle activity that has been caused by hypercapnia, vagal blockade abolishes abdominal muscle activity.[51]

In man at the same levels of ventilation, the abdominal muscles are more active when the stimulus is from hypercapnia, than when the stimulus is hypoxia. There is a close relationship between abdominal muscle activation and pleural pressure increases at end-expiration, indicating that the abdominal muscles are stimulated to contribute more to ventilation by a hypercapnic stimulation.[7]

Hypocapnia

In dogs made hypocapnic, expiratory muscle activity becomes tonic and can be modified by hypoxic stimuli even when spontaneous breathing is not present.[54]

Clinopathological features

In patients with chronic obstructive lung disease, diaphragm action is generally increased but despite this increased activation, abdominal pressure can decrease during inspiration. One explanation of this could be vigorous contraction of the ribcage muscles at the same time,[55] so that the effect of these muscles exceeds the trans-diaphragmatic pressure. However the same decrease could result from a relaxation of the abdominal muscles. In most patients with severe chronic obstructive lung disease, the transversus abdominis, which is the most readily activated of the abdominal muscles, is active during expiration.[56] Bronchoconstriction in patients with COPD causes abdominal muscle recruitment.[57]

Because different stimuli have different effects on the respiratory muscles, it appears that these stimuli cannot have a single pathway through which they affect respiration. The output to the respiratory muscles must receive, at least in part, different inputs: this implies that there may be different strategies available to manipulate ventilation according to the specific pattern of activity that is desired. There is evidence that other stimuli have effects on respiration that are not passed via a "final common pathway". For example, pain can alter resting ventilation but has no apparent effect on the responses to hypoxia.[58] Abdominal muscle activation occurs during general anaesthesia,[59] and may be related to opioid drugs which are known to induce rigidity, by a complex pathway involving several transmitter systems.[60] We recently studied the effects of an opioid, and its reversal with naloxone, during anaesthesia, to assess the relative contributions of opioid and hypercapnia on abdominal muscle activation.

Methods

Seven patients, otherwise healthy, were studied after minor superficial surgery. Passive respiratory system compliance was measured with a large calibrated syringe and a Validyne transducer, while the patients were paralysed with vecuronium. After reversal of the neuromuscular block, anaesthesia was maintained with nitrous oxide and isoflurane and supplemented with a continuous infusion of fentanyl at a rate sufficient to suppress the respiratory rate to between 15 and 20 breath/min. Abdominal EMG was measured with a pair of percutaneous stainless steel wire electrodes. Measurements were made of abdominal

EMG during a control breath, and during airway occlusion at end-inspiration. Airway pressure was measured during occlusion of expiration. To assess expiratory muscle activity, the passive recoil pressure of the respiratory system, calculated from the measured tidal volume and the passive compliance, was subtracted from the occlusion pressure to give the "active" expiratory pressure. Measurements were made during quiet breathing and during stimulation with carbon dioxide, both before and after reversal of the action of the fentanyl with naloxone.

Results

Expiratory occlusion prolonged expiration by about 10%, but the amplitude of the signal in mid-expiration was not altered. Carbon dioxide stimulation had no significant effect on the abdominal EMG nor on the "active" expiratory pressure. After reversal of the opioid effects, abdominal EMG was markedly reduced. This comparison was done at the same PCO_2, using EMG *versus* CO_2 plots for the two conditions. The active pressure generated by the expiratory muscles was reduced , but showed a response to stimulation by CO_2.

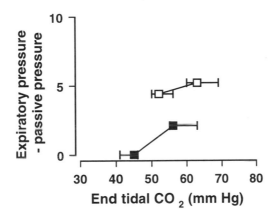

Figure 1. Open symbols, before reversal, closed symbols after reversal with naloxone.

Discussion

We found a good agreement between EMG amplitude and the active expiratory pressure generated by airway occlusion. There was no evidence that this manoeuvre had a reflex effect on the activation of the abdominal muscles. Previous workers have suggested that the effects of morphine could be explained solely by the respiratory depressant effects and the resultant hypercapnia [61] but our results show that in man, the opioid fentanyl has a specific activating effect on the abdominal muscles. Abdominal muscle action is likely to contribute to the changes in abdominal pressure in patients receiving opioid analgesia for pain after upper abdominal surgery.

References

1. Bruce EN, Mitra J, Cherniack NS. Central and peripheral chemoreceptor inputs to phrenic and hypoglossal motoneurons. *J Appl Physiol* 53: 1504-1511, 1982.
2. Newsom Davis J, Plum F. Separation of descending spinal pathways to respiratory motoneurons. *Exp Neurol* 34: 78- 94, 1972.
3. De Troyer A, Estenne M, Ninane V, van Gansbeke D, Gorini M. Transversus abdominis muscle function in humans. *J Appl Physiol* 68: 1010-1016, 1990.
4. Druz WS, Sharp JT. Activity of respiratory muscles in upright and recumbent humans. *J Appl Physiol* 51: 1552-1561, 1982.
5. De Troyer A. Mechanical role of the abdominal muscles in relation to posture. *Respir Physiol* 53: 341-353, 1983.
6. Goldman JM, Lehr RP, Millar AB, Silver JR. An electromyographic study of the abdominal muscles during postural and respiratory maneuvers. *Journal of Neurology, Neurosurgery and Psychiatry* 50: 866-869, 1987.
7. Takasaki Y, Orr D, Popkin J, Xie A, Bradley TD. Effect of hypercapnia and hypoxia on respiratory muscle activation in humans. *J Appl Physiol* 67: 1776-1784, 1989.
8. Wakai Y, Welsh MM, Leevers AM, Road JD. Expiratory muscle activity in the awake and sleeping human during lung inflation and hypercapnia. *J Appl Physiol* 72: 881-887, 1992.
9. Fitzgerald RS. Relationships between tidal volume and phrenic nerbe activity during hypercapnia and hypoxia. *Acta Neurobiol Exp* 33: 419-425, 1973.
10. Fregosi RF, Knuth SL, Ward DK, Bartlett D, Jr. Hypoxia inhibits abdominal expiratory nerve activity. *J Appl Physiol* 63: 211-220, 1987.
11. Garcia A, Cherniack NS. Integrated phrenic nerve activity in hypercapnia and hypoxia. *Anesthesiology* 28: 1029-1035, 1967.
12. Ledlie JF, Pack AI, Fishman AP. Effects of hypercapnia and hypoxia on abdominal expiratory nerve activity. *J Appl Physiol* 55: 1614-1622, 1983.
13. St.John WM. Respiratory neuron responses to hypercapnia and carotid chemoreceptor stimulation. *J Appl Physiol* 51: 816-822, 1981.
14. Rehder K, Sessler AD, Rodarte JR. Regional intrapulmonary gas distribution in awake and anesthetized-paralyzed man. *J Appl Physiol* 42: 391-402, 1977.
15. Grimby G, Bunn J, and Mead J. Relative contribution of ribcage and abdomen to ventilation during exercise. *J Appl Physiol* 24: 159-166, 1968.
16. van der Schans CP, de Jong W, de Vries G, Postma DS, Koeter GH, van der Mark TW. Effect of positive expiratory pressure on breathing pattern on healthy subjects. *Eur Respir J* 6: 60-66, 1993.
17. Koulouris N, Mulvey DA, Laroche CM, Goldstone J, Moxham J, Green M. The effect of posture and abdominal binding on respiratory pressures. *Eur Respir J* 2: 961-965, 1989.
18. Newman SL, Road JD, Grassino A. In vivo length and shortening of canine diaphragm with body postural change. *J Appl Physiol* 60: 661-669, 1985.
19. Henke KG, Sharratt M, Pegelow D, and Dempsey JA. Regulation of end-expiratory lung volume during exercise. *J Appl Physiol* 64: 135-146, 1988.
20. Martin JG, De Troyer A. The behaviour of the abdominal muscles during inspiratory mechanical loading. *Respir Physiol* 50: 63-73, 1982.
21. Abbrecht PH, Rajagopal KR, Kyle RR. Expiratory muscle recruitment during inspiratory

flow-resistive loading and exercise. *Am Rev Respir Dis* 144: 113-120, 1991.

22. Zakynthinos SG, Vassilakopoulos T, Zakynthinos E, Roussos C. Accurate measurement of intrinsic positive end-expiratory pressure: How to detect and correct for expiratory muscle activity. *Eur Respir J* 10: 522-529, 1997.

23. Kyroussis D, Mills GH, Polkey MI et al. Effect of maximum ventilation on abdominal muscle-relaxation rate. *Thorax* 51: 510- 515, 1996.

24. Esau SA, Bye PTP, Pardy RL. Changes in rate of relaxation of sniffs with diaphragmatic fatigue in humans. *J Appl Physiol* 55: 731-735, 1998.

25. Macklem PT, Gross D, Grassino A, Roussos C. Partitioning of inspiratory pressure swings between diaphragm and intercostal/accessory muscles. *J Appl Physiol* 44:200-208, 1978.

26. De Troyer A, Estenne M. Functional anatomy of the respiratory muscles. *Clinics In Chest Medicine* 9: 175-193, 1988.

27. Smith CA, Ainsworth DM, Henderson KS, Dempsey JA. Differential timing of respiratory muscles in response to chemical stimuli in awake dogs. *J Appl Physiol* 66: 392-399, 1989.

28. Koterba AM, Kosch PC, Beech J, Whitlock T. Breathing strategy of the adult horse (equus caballus) at rest. *J Appl Physiol* 64: 337-346, 1988.

29. Gilmartin JJ, Ninane V, De Troyer A. Abdominal muscle use during breathing in the anesthetized dog. *Respir Physiol* 70: 159-171, 1987.

30. Ainsworth DA, Smith CA, Eicker SW, Henderson KS, Dempsey JA. The effects of locomotion on respiratory muscle activity in the awake dog. *Respir Physiol* 78: 145-162, 1989.

31. Ainsworth DA, Smith CA, Eicker SW, Henderson KS, Dempsey JA. The effects of chemical versus locomotory stimuli on respiratory muscle activity in the awake dog. *Respir Physiol* 78: 163-176, 1989.

32. Leevers AM, Road JD. Abdominal muscle-activity during hypercapnia in awake dogs. *J Appl Physiol* 77: 1393-1398, 1994.

33. Warner DO, Joyner MJ, Rehder K. Electrical activation of expiratory muscles increases with time in pentobarbital-anesthetized dogs. *J Appl Physiol* 72:2285-2291, 1992.

34. Bishop B. Reflex control of abdominal muscles during positive-pressure breathing. *J Appl Physiol* 19: 224-232, 1964.

35. De Troyer A, Ninane V. Effect of posture on expiratory muscle use during breathing in the dog. *Respir Physiol* 67: 311-322, 1987.

36. Kelsen SG, Altose MD, Cherniack NS. Interaction of lung volume and chemical drive on respiratory muscle EMG and respiratory timing. *J Appl Physiol* 42: 287-294, 1977.

37. Oliven A, Deal ECj, Kelsen SG, Cherniack NS. Effects of hypercapnia on expiratory and inspiratory muscle activity during expiration. *J Appl Physiol* 59: 1560-1565, 1985.

38. Russell JA, Bishop B. Vagal afferents essential for abdominal muscle activity during lung inflation in cats. *J Appl Physiol* 41: 310-315, 1976.

39. Sibuya M, Homma I. Functional mechanism of expiratory pattern generator. *J Appl Physiol* 67: 199-202, 1989.

40. Fregosi RF. Changes in the neural drive to abdominal expiratory muscles in hemorrhagic hypotension. *Am J Physiol* 266: H2423-H2429, 1994.

41. Watchko JF, Oday TL, Brozanski BS, Guthrie RD. Expiratory abdominal muscle-activity during ventilatory chemostimulation in piglets. *J Appl Physiol* 68: 1343-1349, 1990.

42. Cooke IRC, Soust M, Berger PJ. Differential recruitment of inspiratory muscles in response to chemical drive. *Respir Physiol* 92: 167-181, 1993.

43. van Lunteren E, Haxhiu MA, Cherniack NS, Arnold JS. Rib cage and abdominal expiratory muscle responses to CO_2 and esophageal distension. *J Appl Physiol* 64: 846-853, 1988.

44. Chonan T, Okabe S, Hida W, Izumiyama T, Kikuchi Y, Takishima T. Inhomogeneous response of expiratory muscle-activity to cold block of the ventral medullary surface. *J Appl Physiol* 71: 1723– 1728, 1991.

45. Darian GB, DiMarco AF, Kelsen SG, Supinski GS, Gottfried SB. Effects of progressive hypoxia on parasternal, costal, and crural diaphragm activation. *J Appl Physiol* 66 :2579–2584, 1989.

46. Smith CA, Ainsworth DM, Henderson KS, Dempsey JA. The influence of carotid body chemoreceptors on expiratory muscle activity. *Respir Physiol* 82: 123– 136, 1990.

47. Fregosi RF. Influence of hypoxia and carotid sinus nerve stimulation on abdominal muscle activities in the cat. *J Appl Physiol* 76: 602–609, 1994.

48. Chae LO, Melton JE, Neubauer JA, Edelman NH. Triangularis-sterni and phrenic nerve responses to progressive brain hypoxia. *J Appl Physiol* 72: 1522– 1528, 1992.

49. Nolan PC, Waldrop TG. In vivo and in vitro responses of neurons in the ventrolateral medulla to hypoxia. *Brain Res* 6303: 101– 114, 1993.

50. Smith CA, Ainsworth DM, Henderson KS, Dempsey JA. Differential responses of expiratory muscles to chemical stimuli in awake dogs. *J Appl Physiol* 66: 384– 391, 1989.

51. Yasuma F, Kimoff RJ, Kozar LF, England SJ, Bradley TD, Phillipson EA. Abdominal muscle activation by respiratory stimuli in conscious dogs. *J Appl Physiol* 74: 16– 23, 1993.

52. Smith CA, Engwall MJA, Dempsey JA, Bisgard GE. Effects of specific carotid body and brain hypoxia on respiratory muscle control in the awake goat. *J Physiol Lond* 448: 613– 631, 1992.

53. Denison DM, Morgan MDL, Millar AB. Estimation of regional gas and tissue volumes of the lung in supine man using computed tomography. *Thorax* 41: 620–628, 1986.

54. Horner RL, Kozar LF, Phillipson EA. Tonic respiratory drive in the absence of rhythm generation in the conscious dog. *J Appl Physiol* 76: 671–680, 1998.

55. De Troyer A. Effect of hyperinflation on the diaphragm. *Eur Respir J* 10: 708–713, 1997.

56. Ninane V, Rypens F, Yernault J-C, and De Troyer A. Abdominal muscle use during breathing in patients with chronic airflow obstruction. *Am Rev Respir Dis* 146: 16–21, 1992.

57. Gorini M, Misuri G, Duranti R, Iandelli I, Mancini M, Scano G. Abdominal muscle recruitment and PEEPi during bronchoconstriction in chronic obstructive pulmonary disease. *Thorax* 52: 355–361, 1997.

58. Sarton E, Dahan A, Teppema L et al. Acute pain and central nervous system arousal do not restore impaired hypoxic ventilatory response during sevoflurane sedation. *Anesthesiology* 85: 295–303, 1996.

59. Freund F, Roos A, and Dodd RB. Expiratory activity of the abdominal muscles in man during general anesthesia. *J Appl Physiol* 19: 693–697, 1964.

60. Fu M, Tsen L, Lee T, Lui P, and Chan SHH. Involvement of cerulospinal glutamatergic neurotransmission in fentanyl-induced muscular rigidity in the rat. *Anesthesiology* 87: 1450– 1459, 1997.

61. Howard RS and Sears TA. The effects of opiates on the respiratory activity of thoracic motoneurones in the anaesthetized and decerebrated rabbit. *J Physiol Lond* 437: 181–199, 1991.

Influences of low dose volatile anesthetic agents on ventilatory control in humans: a comparison of the Knill and Leiden studies

Albert Dahan

General considerations

Knowledge on the effects of low- and high-dose volatile anesthetic agents on ventilatory control is import since it influences, at least partly, the clinical management of all patients. It concerns patients during general anesthesia that breathe spontaneously, most postoperative patients after general anesthesia, patients during Monitored Anesthesia Care and patients during labor and dental surgery that require anesthesia and analgesia. Spontaneous respiration during general anesthesia remains popular because of its many advantages: the patient regulates his/her own anesthetic depth, the occurrence of awareness is uncommon, immediate transportation after deep extubation to the Anesthesia Care Unit is possible and there is no need for reversal of muscle relaxants. Disadvantages are respiratory depression, delayed recovery, the risk of upper airway obstruction and aspiration. Some of these may be of lesser importance when using an anesthetic with a low blood-gas partition coefficient that ensures rapid emergence. Sevoflurane and desflurane are examples of new generation halogenated anesthetic agents with such rapid pharmacokinetic characteristics. Lately, the number of patients breathing spontaneously during general anesthesia has increased even more due to the introduction of the Laryngeal Mask Airway.

All inhalational anesthetics agents affect ventilatory control in a dose dependent fashion. It is important to realize that they do so by effects at multiple sites in the body. For example, halothane causes ventilatory depression due to effects at the carotid bodies, within the central nervous system and at the diaphragm and intercostal muscles.

In the late 1970's and early 80's, Richard Knill and colleagues from the University of Western Ontario in London, Ontario, were among the first to study the effects of low concentrations of inhalational anesthetics on the regulation of breathing.[1-5] Their studies led to the still generally accepted conclusion that inhalational anesthetics selectively impair all responses mediated by the peripheral chemoreceptors at subanesthetic concentrations (minimal alveolar concentration [MAC] fractions as low as one-twentieth to one-tenth). Since then, the techniques used by Knill to test hypoxic and hypercapnic responses as well as their results have come under criticism. Recently (from 1992 on), in Leiden, we undertook a series of systematic studies on the influence of low dose anesthetic agents on the ventilatory control system in humans.[6-11]

In this paper, I will discuss the results of the studies of Knill and colleagues and compare them to the relevant studies from Leiden. Richard Knill had much interest in work on the control of breathing and demonstrated this by his intention to analyze some of our data just before he regretfully passed away on January 22, 1995, at the age of 54.

Studies from Knill and colleagues

In a series of three studies, Knill and colleagues investigated the influence of halothane on the chemical control of breathing in volunteers and patients.[1-3] Initially, Knill and Gelb studied the influence of halothane on the ventilatory responses to hypoxia, hypercapnia and doxapram in thirty-three subjects: eight at 0.1 MAC, fifteen at 1.1 MAC and twenty at 2 MAC.[1] Halothane, at 1.1 and 2 MAC, totally abolished the hypoxic response and nearly abolished the response to doxapram. At 0.1 MAC the response to hypoxia was reduced by more than 70% while the slope of the hyperoxic ventilatory-carbon dioxide (V_I-PCO_2) response was not affected. An interesting observation was that at anesthetic halothane concentrations, hypoxia (especially against a background of hypercapnia) caused a reduction in V_I (by 30 % or more) rather than an increase. At this point, we have to keep in mind that hypoxia was induced by rebreathing a gas mixture from a balloon for about 10 min, and therefore, that the measured ventilatory response was a carotid body response contaminated by the central depressant effects of sustained (i.e. > 3 min) hypoxia on V_I. Hypercapnia was induced by rebreathing a hyperoxic gas mixture from a 4 to 6 liter balloon. This method yields results that are often difficult to interpret.[12]

Additionally, Knill and Clement studied the wash-in of 0.15 to 0.30 % inspired halothane on steady-state hypoxic ventilation, in 6 subjects.[2] Upon exposure to halothane, hypoxia-driven V_I decreased promptly to about 75 % of control at 30 s and to about 60% at 1 min of wash-in. To estimate brain and carotid body halothane concentrations a simple model was used for halothane uptake from the lung, based on standard pharmacokinetic principles. Knill and Clement estimated that at 30 s of wash-in, brain halothane tension was less than 2% of end-tidal while the carotid body halothane tension was 70 % of end-tidal. At 60 s of wash-in these values were 10% and 90%, respectively. They concluded that "the evidence favors the carotid bodies as major site of desensitization of the peripheral chemoreflex pathway by subanesthetic halothane".[2]

In a third series of experiment Knill and Clement gathered further proof for a selective effect of subanesthetic halothane at the site of the peripheral chemoreceptors of the carotid bodies. In this study acute metabolic acidosis was induced by infusing L-arginine hydrochloride in 14 volunteers. Isocapnic ventilatory-$[H^+]_a$ responses were determined in hyperoxia, normoxia and hypoxia in the awake state and during inhalation of 0.1 and 1 MAC halothane. Their results imply that acute, moderate metabolic acidosis increases V_I mainly through stimulation of the peripheral chemoreceptors. In normoxia, they observed a reduction of the V_I-$[H^+]_a$ response by 60% and 80% at 0.1 and 1 MAC halothane, respectively. Furthermore, the ventilatory response to carotid body-mediated $[H^+]$-hypoxia interaction was markedly reduced at both halothane concentrations.

After having having studied halothane, Knill and colleagues proceeded their research with studies on enflurane and isoflurane in 23 and 12 subjects, respectively.[4,5] The results of the hypoxic studies were in agreement with their earlier findings on halothane. However, the hyperoxic CO_2 rebreathing tests were not uniform: no effect of 0.1 MAC isoflurane on the V_I-PCO_2 response slope, but a reduction of 25% of the response slope at 0.1 MAC enflurane.

The results of the above studies lead to the conclusion that all halogenated anesthetic agents at subanesthetic concentrations cause "the effective loss of peripheral chemoreflex-mediated functions in the presence of hypoxemia, [which means] not only loss of physiological defenses but loss of useful clinical signs". This statement was made by Knill and Gelb in an editorial in the journal Anesthesiology in 1982.[13] These statements were of special importance in the days that "arterial oxygen saturation could not be monitored continuously in an economical and reliable way".[13] Something anesthesiologist today possibly cannot imagine. However, also today these statements retain their importance for large groups of perioperative patients (see above).

Comparison of studies

In Leiden, we started studying the influence of halothane on ventilatory control in 1992, after a six year delay. Initially we studied the influence of 0.076% and 0.15% inspired halothane (equivalent to 0.05 and 0.1 MAC) on the ventilatory response to acute hypoxia and the dynamic ventilatory response to carbon dioxide in 9 male subjects.[6] We used the "Dynamic End-Tidal Forcing" technique to apply steps in CO_2 and steps into (and out of) hypoxia.[12] With respect to the CO_2 response, this technique enables us to separate the ventilatory response into a fast, peripheral component and a slow, central component. With respect to the hypoxic response, this technique enables us to separate the carotid body response from the central depressive effects of hypoxia on V_I. We observed a reduction of the acute hypoxic response at 0.1 MAC halothane by more than 70 %. There was no effect of halothane on the central CO_2 sensitivity. However, the peripheral CO_2 sensitivity was 50 % of control at 0.1 MAC halothane. In a second study of halothane, we tested the effect of halothane sedation (0.15 MAC) on the ventilatory response into and out of sustained (that is, 20 min) isocapnic hypoxia in fourteen subjects.[7] The major findings from that study were: 1) at 20 min of hypoxia mean V_I was not different from pre-hypoxic mean baseline V_I; 2) at the termination of hypoxia, mean V_I showed an undershoot below mean pre-hypoxic V_I; 3) in 2 subjects several periods of central apnea occurred at the termination of hypoxia.

All of these findings are in close agreement with those of Knill and colleagues and point towards a selective effect of subanesthetic halothane on the peripheral chemoreflex loop as well as a synergistic interaction between halothane and sustained hypoxia on V_I. This is important to clinicians caring for a patient during anesthesia or monitored anesthesia care: when hypoxic for periods longer than 3 to 5 min, the patient will reduce his/her ventilation, despite hypercapnia. This stands in sharp contrast to the brisk hyperventilatory response to asphyxia (hypoxia combined with hypercapnia) when awake.

In a series of four different protocols we studied the influences of subanesthetic isoflurane on ventilatory control.[8,9] In twenty-one subjects, we studied ventilatory responses to acute and sustained hypoxia (Study I), the dynamic ventilatory response to CO_2 (Study II), the response to isoflurane wash-in during sustained isocapnic hypoxia (Study III), and the influence of extraneous input in the form of audio and visual stimulation on isoflurane-induced depression of the acute hypoxic response (Study IV). The findings of Studies I and

II were similar to the findings of Knill et al.[5] on isoflurane and our earlier findings with halothane. Study III was designed to locate the site of action of subanesthetic isoflurane. After at least 15 min of isocapnic hypoxia and steady-state V_I had been reached, a step in end-tidal isoflurane tension from 0 to 1 mmHg (~0.1 MAC) was performed within 4 to 6 breaths. Within 30 s of exposure to isoflurane, V_I decreased from 153% to 107% of pre-hypoxic baseline V_I. In cooperation with Knill, we analyzed the data, using a model similar to that used for halothane,[2] and concluded that isoflurane at 0.1 MAC affects ventilatory control at the site of the peripheral chemoreceptors of the carotid bodies. In fact, our results with isoflurane were identical to those of Knill and Clement on halothane.[2] Study IV showed that activation of behavioral control of breathing via stimulation of auditory and visual central pathways inflated the isoflurane-reduced acute hypoxic response. I consider the fact that the response became identical to control as coincidental. The latter study shows the importance of controlling background stimuli when studying chemical control of breathing.

Finally, we studied the influence of two newly introduced anesthetics: sevoflurane and desflurane.[10,11] Results from these studies were surprising. Sevoflurane, at 0.23 end-tidal % (~ 0.13 MAC) reduced the acute hypoxic response by 30%. However, EEG-monitored arousal from administration of painful stimuli, did not affect the sevoflurane-induced depression of the hypoxic response. This finding is in contrast with those with isoflurane and audio/visual stimulation (see above) and indicates the complexity of the interaction of anesthesia, sedation, pain, arousal and behavioral stimuli on the chemical control of breathing. This topic remains poor understood and deserves further study.

Desflurane, at 0.1 MAC, did not reduce the V_I normocapnic hypoxic response, but did reduce the response in terms of tidal volume. Furthermore, the V_I response to asphyxia was reduced by about a third. This seems to contrast with the belief that, with respect to the control of breathing, all halogenated anesthetic behave in a similar fashion. However, the translation of the hypoxic-hypercapnic interaction into V_I at the carotid bodies does not involve a fundamentally different mechanism from the hypoxic response at (near)-normocapnia. The observation that the response to asphyxia is affected by 0.1 MAC desflurane then indicates that the carotid bodies are affected in a similar fashion as during inhalation of the other anesthetic agents. Possibly, other properties of desflurane (for example, an increase of sympathetic activity) interacting with acute hypoxia, may have counteracted the depression of the carotid bodies in terms of V_I.

Conclusions

Despite differences in techniques, the results obtained from the Leiden studies are in close agreement with those of Knill's group. While the rebreathing techniques used by Knill are considered no longer appropriate for drug research since they yield results that may be difficult to interpret and quantitatively not always in agreement with steady-state techniques,[12] the others (ref. 2 and 3) are clearly not inferior to the sophisticated technique used in Leiden. Taken into account the above, I conclude, without any reserve, that the statements made by Knill and Gelb in 1982 still hold good.[13]

It is of interest to note that the close agreement between the study on the influence of halothane on the V_I-$[H^+]_a$ response and the dynamic response to CO_2, using the dynamic end-tidal forcing technique, strongly support the overall validity of the dynamic end-tidal forcing technique in studying ventilatory control in humans.

Acknowledgement: This paper was made possible by a grant from Datex-Engstrom BV.

References
1. Knill RL, Gelb AW. Ventilatory responses to hypoxia and hypercapnia during halothane sedation and anesthesia. *Anesthesiology* 49: 244-251, 1978.
2. Knill RL, Clement JL. Site of selective action of halothane on the peripheral chemoreflex loop pathway in humans. *Anesthesiology* 61: 121-126, 1984.
3. Knill RL, Clement JL. Ventilatory responses to acute metabolic acidemia in humans awake, sedated, and anesthetized with halothane. *Anesthesiology* 62: 745-753, 1985.
4. Knill RL, Manninen PH, Clement JL. Ventilation and chemoreflexes during enflurane sedation and anaesthesia in man. *Can Anaesth Soc J* 26: 353-360, 1979.
5. Knill RL, Kieraszewicz HT, Dodgson BG, Celemnt JL. Chemical regulation of ventilation during isoflurane sedation and anaesthesia in humans. *Can Anaesth Soc J* 30: 607-614, 1983.
6. Dahan A, van den Elsen M, Berkenbosch A, DeGoede J, Olievier I, van Kleef J, Bovill J. Effects of subanesthetic halothane on the ventilatory response to hypercapnia and acute hypoxia in healthy volunteers. *Anesthesiology* 80: 727-738, 1994.
7. Dahan A, van den Elsen M, Berkenbosch A, DeGoede J, Olievier I, Burm A, van Kleef J. Influence of a subanesthetic concentration of halothane on the ventilatory response to step changes into and out of sustained isocapnic hypoxia in healthy volunteers. *Anesthesiology* 81: 850-859, 1994.
8. van den Elsen M, Dahan A, DeGoede J, Berkenbosch A, van Kleef J. Influences of subanesthetic isoflurane on ventilatory control in humans. *Anesthesiology* 83: 478-490, 1995.
9. van den Elsen M, Dahan A, Berkenbosch A, DeGoede J, van Kleef J, Olievier I. Does subanesthetic isoflurane affect the ventilatory response to acute isocapnic hypoxia in healthy volunteers? *Anesthesiology* 81: 860-867, 1994.
10. Sarton E, Dahan A, Teppema L, van den Elsen M, Olofsen E, Berkenbosch A, van Kleef J. Acute pain and central nervous system arousal do not restore impaired hypoxic ventilatory response during sevoflurane sedation. *Anesthesiology* 85: 295-303, 1996.
11. Dahan A, Sarton E, van den Elsen M, van Kleef J, Teppema L, Berkenbosch A. Ventilatory response to hypoxia in humans: influences of subanesthetic desflurane. *Anesthesiology* 85: 60-68, 1996.
12. Dahan A. The ventilatory response to carbon dioxide and oxygen in man: methods and implications. PhD Thesis. Leiden University, Leiden, 1990.
13. Knill RL, Gelb AW. Peripheral chemoreceptors during anesthesia: are the watchdogs sleeping? *Anesthesiology* 57: 151-152, 1982.

Cardiovascular and pulmonary interactions in pharmacokinetics

Jette A. Kuipers and Fred Boer

The fate of drugs in the body is dependent on the physical transport processes in the body. These transport processes are initiated by the flow of blood in the greater and lesser circulation by which the drug is carried to the organs and tissues, where the drug is taken up by active and passive transport mechanisms. The blood flow therefore plays an important role in the initial distribution of drugs and the extend of distribution of the drug within a certain time frame. The influence of the hemodynamic system and the lungs can be modeled, using pharmacokinetic models.

Influence of cardiac output and pulmonary uptake on pharmacokinetics
The term 'pharmacokinetics' refers to prediction of the time-dependent concentrations of a substance in a living system. Determination of dosing schedules for anesthetics depends not only on the pharmacokinetics of the drug, but also on the physical condition of the patient and thus on the relationship between physiology of the patient and drug pharmacokinetics. The pharmacokinetics of all anesthetics have been thoroughly investigated. Furthermore, the circulation of all patients under anesthesia is well monitored. Despite this, however, the interaction between the drug and the patients physiology and *vice versa* has been studied only to a small extent. It may be worthwhile to study this interaction, considering the importance of the circulation for the distribution of drugs in the body.

One of the important interactions between pharmacokinetics and circulatory physiology is the affect of cardiac output on the distribution of drugs in the body.[1] Cardiac output was found to largely determine the intercompartmental clearance (i.e. distribution clearance) of alfentanil in humans.[2] Not only cardiac output will change the distribution of drugs in the body. Changes in cardiac output will usually be accompanied by changes in regional blood flows, changing the flow allocation over the organs and tissues. Thus a decrease of the cardiac output can cause a decreased hepatic blood flow. Especially for drugs with a high hepatic extraction ratio the blood flow through the liver is very important. Since the blood flow through the liver is generally considered to be approximately 25% of the cardiac output,[3] for these drugs the elimination clearance is strongly dependent on cardiac output. When cardiac output is larger, an increased elimination clearance can result in a decreased duration of action. For sheep it has been shown that an increased cardiac output results in a decreased duration of propofol anesthesia, analyzing propofol kinetics with a physiological model.[4]

The interaction between pharmacokinetics and circulatory physiology also plays an important role in the immediate availability of a drug. The lungs, intertwined between the intravenous injection site and the systemic circulation, can retain significant amounts of the injected dose, thus decreasing the arterial concentrations immediately after injection. This first-pass effect is particularly significant for the basic amines, to which many anesthetics belong. Drugs such as lidocaine,[5,6] propranolol, [7] fentanyl[8] and meperidine[8] all undergo significant first-pass uptake in the lungs. As a result, only 20% to 40% of the dose of these drugs enters the systemic circulation immediately after intravenous administration. Usually the drug retained in the lungs is gradually released from the lung tissue and the lungs seldom have a significant metabolic capacity for the drug. The lungs therefore essentially acts as a capacitor, limiting the rate at which the injected dose enters the systemic circulation. This will play a role in the early pharmacokinetics of these drugs and possible influence the time to onset of pharmacological action.[9]

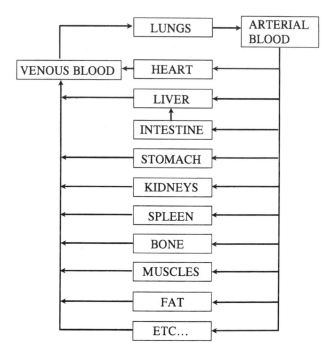

Figure 1. This figure shows an example of a physiological model. In this model, blood from the arterial blood pool supplies the various organs and tissues of arterial blood. Blood from the various organs and tissues is then gathered in the venous blood pool. Venous blood passes the lungs and then enters again the arterial blood pool. This is a simple physiological model. The more organs, sometimes even different cell types in the organs, and tissue groups the model contains, the better it describes what actually happens, but the more difficult it is to obtain all parameters.

Compartmental models

The pharmacokinetics of drugs can be described by pharmacokinetic models. Usually these models are derived from the mathematical description of concentration-time curves, two- or three exponential equations, which are translated into so-called structural models, the two- and three-compartment models. These structural models consist of a central compartment by which the drug enters the system and from which the drug will eventually be eliminated, assuming that the drug is immediately and completely mixed in this central compartment. This central compartment is connected to one or two "peripheral" or "deep" compartments that function as sinks for the drug. These models are very useful to describe the long-term distribution and elimination in the body. Limitations of these compartmental models for the interpretation of bolus kinetics are that they give a poor description of intravascular mixing[10] during the first minutes after injection, before complete mixing of the drug in the blood has occurred, and of lung kinetics including first-pass lung uptake.[9,11] Furthermore the model cannot include directly the effect of a change in cardiac output in the model. Cardiac output as a independent cofactor in a population approach of compartmental modeling does not foreclose the problems that arise from the assumption of initial complete mixing. Therefore, if the initial mixing and transit through the lungs are to be described, the model is of limited value.

Physiological models

A more realistic approach to the study of the influence of the circulation on the distribution of drugs in the body is to derive a physiological model that emulates, as far as possible, what actually happens in the body (see figure 1). Such a model may comprise a number of perfusion-limited compartments, each defined in terms of volume, blood-flow, and apparent tissue:blood partition coefficient λ_{TB}. The greater the number of identifiable compartments, the closer the model may be expected to emulate drug disposition in patients. An advantage of such models lies in their ability to account for hemodynamic changes, such as altered cardiac output or flow re-allocation. They have one great drawback: numerical values must be assigned to all the parameters, and this may present an insuperable difficulty.[12] It is impossible to determine all these parameters in one animal, let alone that this is impossible in human research. For this reason most parameters for physiological models are first determined in small animals and then scaled up to man. Parameters must be estimated from the animal studies, equilibrium dialysis of tissues taken from other patients and from literature studies of hemodynamics. The model therefore does hardly allow for individualization, beside on the basis of general descriptors like age and weight.

Recirculatory models

A recirculatory model is a compromise between a compartmental model and a physiological model. The recirculatory model was first described by Krejcie et al.[13] The model consists of compartments in series and in parallel (see figure 2). The compartments between the right atrial point of injection and the arterial sampling site are considered to present the central circulation and tissues. The compartments between the arterial sampling site and the right

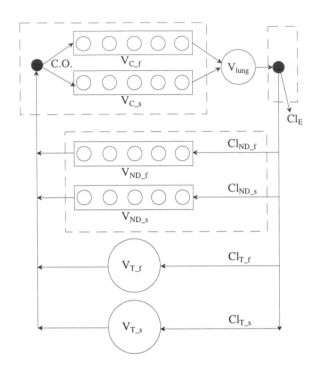

Figure 2. The recirculatory pharmacokinetic model used for analysis of indocyanine green (ICG) and simultaneously injected alfentanil (modified from Krejcie et al.[13]). In this case the simultaneously injected alfentanil has considerable lung-uptake (V_{lung}) and a slow (V_{T_s}) and a fast (V_{T_f}) peripheral tissue compartment. The parts in the dashed boxes represent the recirculatory model for ICG, the intra vascular part of the model. These intravascular compartments are represented by a rectangle with five compartments, but the actual number of compartments may vary and has no physiological background, the concept of these compartments in series is only used to be able to describe the data properly. The intra vascular model consists of: a central part, receiving all of cardiac output, divided in a slow (V_{c_s}) and a fast (V_{c_f}) central compartment and a peripheral part, divided in a slow (V_{ND_s}) and a fast (V_{ND_f}) peripheral compartment. The simultaneous injected alfentanil distributes into organs and tissue and therefore three extravascular compartments are added to the intravascular ICG model. The sum of the peripheral clearances equals the cardiac output.

arterial injection point are considered to represent the peripheral circulation and tissues. The model furthermore consists of the intravascular compartments, identified by using an intravascular marker indocyanine green (ICG) by fitting the intravascular model to the ICG data. Once the intravascular model has been identified, this is used to identify the model for the drug, by including tissue compartments. To allow modeling of a drug the study must therefore be performed by injecting the study drug together with ICG. The recirculatory model is capable of describing the initial mixing of drug in blood, accounting for the first-pass peak concentration. The model was capable to describe the effect of changing of cardiac output on the pharmacokinetics of alfentanil in pigs [Kuipers et al, in press]. Furthermore the influence of lung uptake can be readily incorporated into the model, by including a pulmonary volume of distribution.

Conclusions

As described above, the circulation and the lungs have a significant effect on the fate of drugs in the body, particularly during initial distribution during the first minutes after drug injection. Especially for drugs with a fast onset of effect, such as muscle relaxants and many other anesthetic drugs, initial distribution and availability are very important. For some muscle relaxants it is well-known that cardiac output determines the onset time, often before complete mixing is obtained. Because classical compartmental models are incapable of describing initial distribution before complete mixing is obtained, the relationship between the pharmacokinetics and the pharmacodynamics can only be described after complete mixing. Classical compartmental models give a very poor description of pulmonary first-pass uptake and neglect the decreased availability the first minutes after intravenous injection. In anesthesia, where often drugs with a fast onset of effect are used and availability of drugs plays a very important role, classical compartmental models to describe pharmacokinetics seem to have some limitations. An option is to describe the interaction between physiology and pharmacokinetics with physiological models. These models approach best what really happens with the drug after injection. However, these models have shown to be impossible to determine in the individual patient and therefore cannot be used for individualization. The recirculatory model appears to be a good alternative, since the parameters can be determined in the individual patient which makes them useful for individualization. They overcome two of the major shortcoming of the classical compartmental models since they are capable of describing the initial mixing and the transit through the lungs.

References

1. Upton RN, Huang YF. Influence of cardiac output, injection time and injection volume on the initial mixing of drugs with venous blood after i.v. bolus administration to sheep. *Br J Anaesth* 70: 333-338, 1993.
2. Henthorn TK, Krejcie TC, Avram MJ. The relationship between alfentanil distribution kinetics and cardiac output. *Clin Pharmacol Ther* 52: 190-196, 1992.
3. Greenway CV, Stark RD. Hepatic vascular bed. *Physiol Rev* 51: 23-65, 1971.
4. Ludbrook GL, Upton RN. A physiological model of induction of anaesthesia with propofol in sheep. 2. Model analysis and implications for dose requirements. *Br J Anaesth* 79: 505-513, 1997.
5. Jorfeldt L, Lewis DH, Löfström JB, Post C. Lung uptake of lidocaine in healthy volunteers. *Acta Anaesthesiol Scand* 23: 567-574, 1979.
6. Jorfeldt L, Lewis DH, Löfström JB, Post C. Lung uptake of lidocaine in man as influenced by anaesthesia, mepivacaine infusion or lung insufficiency. *Acta Anaesthesiol Scand* 27: 5-9, 1983.

7.   Geddes DM, Nesbitt K, Traill T, Blackburn JP. First pass uptake of ^{14}C-propranolol by the lung. *Thorax* 34: 810-813, 1979.

8.   Roerig DL, Kotrly KJ, Vucins EJ, Ahlf SB, Dawson CA, Kampine JP. First pass uptake of fentanyl, meperidine, and morphine in the human lung. *Anesthesiology* 67: 466-472, 1987.

9.   Roerig DL, Kotrly KJ, Dawson CA, Ahlf SB, Gualtieri JF, Kampine JP. First-pass uptake of verapamil, diazepam, and thiopental in the human lung. *Anesth Analg* 69: 461-466, 1989.

10.   Henthorn TK, Avram MJ, Krejcie TC. Intravascular mixing and drug disposition: The concurrent disposition of thiopental and indocyanine green. *Clin Pharmacol Ther* 45:5 6-65,1989.

11.   Chiou WL. Potential pitfalls in the conventional pharmacokinetic studies: Effects of the initial mixing of drug in blood and the pulmonary first-pass elimination. *J Pharmacokin Biopharm* 7: 527-536, 1979.

12.   Hull CJ. How far can we go with compartmental models? *Anesthesiology* 72:3 99-402, 1990.

13.   Krejcie TC, Henthorn TK, Niemann CU, Klein C, Gupta DK, Gentry WB, Shanks CA, Avram MJ. Recirculatory pharmacokinetic models of markers of blood, extracellular fluid and total body water administered concomitantly. *J Pharmacol Exp Ther* 278: 1050-1057, 1996.

Pharmacokinetic-pharmacodynamic modeling of sevoflurane-induced respiratory depression in the cat

Erik Olofsen, Albert Dahan, Luc Teppema, Elise Sarton, Cees Olievier

Introduction

Sevoflurane, like the other inhalational anesthetics, exhibits ventilatory depressant effects; during inhalation, the ventilatory controller responds less intense but faster to steps in the P_{et,CO_2} [1]. In this paper, we propose a dynamic model of the changes in baseline ventilation ($\dot{V}_{insp}$), while keeping P_{et,CO_2} and P_{et,O_2} constant.

Methods

The experimental setup has been previously described in detail[2]. Briefly, one cat was lightly anesthetized with α-chloralose-urethane. A control system clamps the P_{et,CO_2} and P_{et,O_2} at about 6 and 15.5 kPa respectively, independent of changes in ventilation by automatically adjusting the inspiratory concentrations. The pharmacokinetics and pharmacodynamics of sevoflurane were investigated by performing step-wise changes in $P_{et,sevo}$ (target values of 1 vol% (run 1) and 1.5 vol% (runs 2-4)), with a duration of approximately 15 minutes. Mathematical models, as described in the next section were fit to the data using nonlinear regression.

The pharmacokinetic-pharmacodynamic model

Pharmacokinetic-pharmacodynamic modelling is the compilation of available knowledge and appropriate assumptions in a mathematical model and the simultaneous estimation of the model parameters from measured responses caused by the administration of a drug. In some cases, it may not be necessary to measure the concentration of the drug in the blood. In this study, the end-tidal volume fraction of sevoflurane was measured, and the pharmacokinetic part of the model needs only describe the relationship between the end-tidal concentration and the brain concentration.

Assuming flow-limited drug disposition in the brain, which is reasonable for lipophylic drugs, the brain can be approximated by one compartment, described by

$$\lambda_{t,b} V_{br} \frac{dC_{br}(t)}{dt} = \dot{Q}_{br}(C_{art}(t) - C_{br}(t)) \tag{1}$$

where t is time, C_{art} is the concentration in the arterial blood, C_{br} is the concentration in the brain, $\lambda_{t,b}$ is the tissue-blood partition coefficient, V_{br} is the volume of the brain compartment and $\dot{Q}_{br}$ is the cerebral blood flow. C_{art} is given by the product of $P_{et,sevo}$ and the blood-gas partition coefficient, assuming that arterial partial pressure equals end-tidal pressure. Note that by defining $k_{e0} = \dot{Q}_{br}/(\lambda_{t,b}V_{br})$, this model is equivalent with the so-called effect compartment which is well-known in the PK-PD literature.

The pharmacodynamic part of the model describes the relationship between the brain concentration and the measured effect, in our case ventilation. An immediate, non-linear relationship can suitably be described by the (inhibitory) sigmoid-emax model, also called the Hill equation:

$$\dot{V}_{insp} = E_{min} + (E_{max} - E_{min}) \cdot \frac{C_e^\gamma(t)}{C_e^\gamma(t) + C_{e,50}^\gamma} = \frac{\dot{V}_{max}}{1 + (C_e(t)/C_{e,50})^\gamma} \tag{2}$$

where $\dot{V}_{insp}$ denotes inspired ventilation, minimal effect $E_{min} = \dot{V}_{max}$ is baseline $\dot{V}_{insp}$, maximal effect $E_{max} = \dot{V}_{min}$ is $\dot{V}_{insp}$ at maximal depression; since sevoflurane can completely block ventilation, $\dot{V}_{min}$ is defined to be zero. Furthermore $C_e = C_{br}$ is the effect-site concentration, $C_{e,50}$ is the concentration which results in 50% of maximal effect and γ is a steepness parameter. An analog combination of the above effect compartment and Hill equation was proposed in 1979 by Sheiner *et al.* to describe the relation between the arterial concentration of the muscle relaxant *d*-tubocurarine and the resulting muscle relaxation[3]. This PK-PD model has been applied to the depression of ventilation due to morphine and fentanyl[4], and to describe many other effects of drugs, *e.g.* the EEG[5].

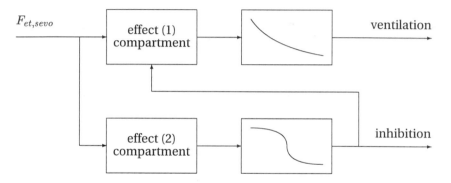

Figure 1: *Schematic diagram of the extended PK-PD model*

An extension of the model to enable it to describe the characteristics of more complex responses (see results), is having one of the parameters dependent on the sevoflurane concentration. For example, by decreasing the value of k_{e0} when $F_{et,sevo}$ is high, $\dot{V}_{insp}$ will slowly return to baseline and subsequently faster when $F_{et,sevo}$ is low. An alternative is to split k_{e0} into k_{in} and k_{out} like has been proposed for the class of "indirect response models"[6], so that:

$$\frac{dC_{br}(t)}{dt} = k_{in} - inh \cdot k_{out} \cdot C_{br}(t) = k_{e0} \cdot (C_{art}(t) - inh \cdot C_{br}(t)) \tag{3}$$

where inh is an inhibition factor. This has about the same effects as inhibiting k_{e0}, but C_{br} is still sensitive to changes in C_{art}, and there is an additional rise in C_{br} at the moment k_{out} is inhibited, resulting in a secondary decrease in $\dot{V}_{insp}$. To model a lag and non-linear relationship between end-tidal concentration and inhibition factor, a second effect compartment and Hill equation need to be incorporated. The complete model is shown in figure 1.

Results

Figure 2 shows two representative responses of $\dot{V}_{insp}$ to step-wise changes in $F_{et,sevo}$. The response in the left panel was satisfactorily fit by the Sheiner model. From a wash-out

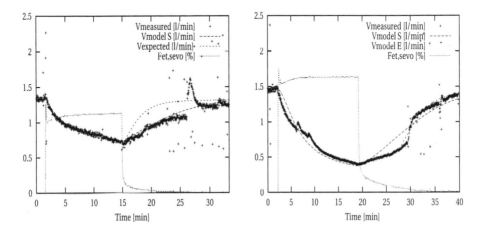

Figure 2: *Left panel: An example of the ventilatory response (run 1) to a step in the sevoflurane concentration of 1%, with a fit of the Sheiner model, and a prediction based on literature (see text). Right panel: An example of a more complex response (run 3) to a step of 1.5%, with fits of the Sheiner and the extended models.*

curve of sevoflurane from the brain of a rat[7], with an inspiratory sevoflurane concentration of 3%, a prediction of the return to baseline was made. The difference between the prediction and the measured ventilation suggests that k_{e0} contains a pharmacodynamic component. In the right panel, a more complex response is shown. We observed the following characteristics: there is an immediate response to changes in the $F_{et,sevo}$; approximately halfway the decline, the rate of fall becomes faster; the return to baseline at the end of the input step is very slow for about ten minutes, and is very fast for the next few minutes. The extended model where k_{out} is inhibited is perfectly capable of describing these characteristics, except the sudden fast return, where its description is reasonable.

In figure 3 the fits of the Sheiner and extended models to two consecutive responses to steps of different magnitudes are shown together with blood pressure. The Sheiner model was allowed to fit only the first response, so that it describes it as well as the extended model. The extended model fits the consecutive responses well. The slow return to baseline of $\dot{V}_{insp}$ seems not to be related to blood pressure, indicating that the inhibitance of k_{out} is a pharmacodynamic phenomenon, residing in the ventilatory controller.

In table 1, numerical values of the estimated parameters of the model fits as shown in

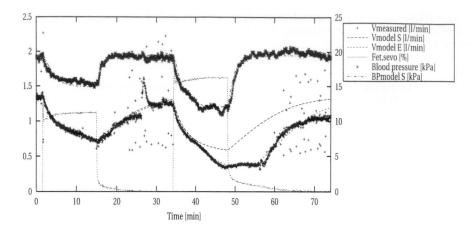

Figure 3: *Two consecutive responses (runs 1+2), fit by the Sheiner and extended models. For comparison, also shown is the blood pressure; for fun, it is fit by the Sheiner model.*

the figures are summarized. Note that γ_2 is very high, suggesting a threshold effect. Because of this, the other parameters of the second effect compartment and Hill equation, $k_{e0,2}$ and $F_{et,50,2}$, control the instants at which the secondary depression and sudden recovery occur. So, to validate the predictive power of these parameters it is necessary to fit two or more consecutive responses. In figure 4 the fit of the extended model is shown, from which it appears that the prediction is reasonable.

	Run 1	Run 3,S	Run3,E	Run 1+2	Run 3+4	BP
$\dot{V}/BP_{max}$	1.37	1.46	1.42	1.32	1.45	19.4
$F_{et,50}$	1.09	0.73	1.90	1.20	2.48	2.09
k_{e0}	0.156	0.102	0.312	0.168	0.450	0.534
γ	1.05	1.76	1.16	1.03	0.96	1.90
inh_{max}			0.25	0.04	0.15	
$F_{et,50,2}$			0.67	0.72	0.65	
$k_{e0,2}$			0.090	0.081	0.102	
γ_2			72	1000	20	

Table 1: *Results of the model fits as shown in the figures. Parameters are explained in the text, except inh_{max} which is the maximal factor with which k_{out} is decreased from k_{e0}; subscript 2 refers to the second effect compartment and Hill equation.*

Discussion

We propose a dynamic model of the respiratory depression induced by sevoflurane. It is an extension of the classical Sheiner model. By inhibiting k_{out} (see eq. (3)), it is capable of describing complex characteristics of ventilatory responses. Since the effect-site concentration C_e (see eq. (2)) does not follow the wash-out curve of sevoflurane from the brain, C_e can not be equal to the sevoflurane C_{br}, but might be related to another chemical substance, such as a neurotransmitter or neuromodulator.

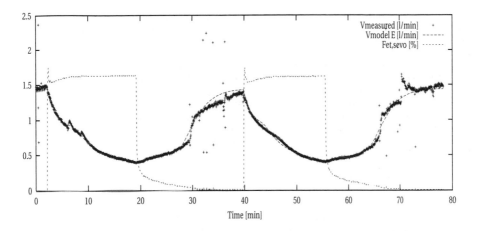

Figure 4: *Two consecutive responses (runs 3+4), fit by the extended model.*

Inhalational anesthetics are known to enhance $GABA_A$-mediated inhibition in the mammalian central nervous system. One of the mechanisms appears to be the inhibition of the catabolism of GABA, leading to elevated GABA concentrations at inhibitory synapses[8]. The effects of GABA in the respiratory network are decreased respiratory motor amplitude and frequency[9]. Sevoflurane also decreases the sensitivity of the central and peripheral chemoreceptors[1]. The reduced input from the chemoreceptor might cause $GABA_A$-mediated inhibition of the respiratory rhythm generator. In our model, C_{br} might reflect the GABA concentration, and k_{in} the GABA production rate.

The proposed model belongs to the class of indirect response models, when the effect of a drug related to the one that is administered is measured[6]. Such models have been applied successfully to describe tolerance, see *e.g.* Wakelkamp[10]. In our case, k_{in} and k_{out} are stimulated and inhibited respectively, describing intensification instead of tolerance. Parameter γ_2, which describes the steepness of the effect of sevoflurane on the inhibition factor has quite a big value. The mechanism of this threshold phenomenon is unclear.

It must be emphasized that different models with the same number of parameters can also approximate the measured data. It is difficult to assess the validity of models like this with which we try to peek into a black box such as the central nervous system without measuring the concentration of neurotransmitters. Experiments, in which the ventilation and other life signs are simultaneously measured, or experiments with anesthetics with different mechanisms of action, may increase the explanatory value of the model.

Acknowledgement: This paper was made possible by a grant from Datex-Engstrom B.V.

References

1. Teppema LJSM, Sarton EY, Olievier CN, Dahan A. Effects of sevoflurane on the dynamics of the ventilatory CO_2 response in lightly anesthetized cats. In: *Proceedings of the Canadian conference on modelling and control of ventilation (VIITH Oxford conference)*, Huntsville, Ontario, Canada, 1997.

2. Berkenbosch A, Teppema LJSM, Olievier CN, Dahan A. Influences of morphine on the ven-

tilatory response to isocapnic hypoxia. *Anesthesiology* 86:1342–1349, 1997.

3. Sheiner LB, Stanski DR, Vozeh S, Miller RD, Ham J. Simultaneous modeling of pharmacokinetics and pharmacodynamics: application to d-tubocurarine. *Clin Pharmacol Ther* 25: 358–371, 1979.

4. Bragg P, Zwass MS, Lau M, Fisher DM. Opioid pharmacodynamics in neonatal dogs: differences between morphine and fentanyl. *J Appl Physiol* 79:1519–1524, 1995.

5. Scott JC, Cooke JE, Stanski DR. Electroencephalographic quantitation of opioid effect: comparative pharmacodynamics of fentanyl and sufentanil. *Anesthesiology* 74:34–43, 1991.

6. Krzyzanski W, Jusko WJ. Mathematical formalism for the properties of four basic models of indirect responses. *J Pharmacokin Biopharm* 25:107–123, 1997.

7. Stern RC, Towler SC, White PF, Evers AS. Elimination kinetics of sevoflurane from blood, brain and adipose tissue in the rat. *Anesth Analg* 71:658–664, 1990.

8. Tanelian DL, Kosek P, Mody I, MacIver MB. The role of the $GABA_A$ receptor/chloride channel complex in anesthesia. *Anesthesiology* 78:757–776, 1993.

9. Bonham AC. Neurotransmitters in the CNS control of breathing. *Respir Physiol* 101:219–230, 1995.

10. Wakelkamp M, Alván G, Gabrielsson J, Paintaud G. Pharmacodynamic modeling of furosemide tolerance after multiple intravenous administration. *Clin Pharmacol Ther* 60:75–88, 1996.

An empirical model of the dynamic ventilatory response to hypoxia in normal subjects

Patricia M. Warren and Peter K. Wraith

Introduction

In 1992, Berkenbosch and colleagues[1] reported that the peripheral chemoreceptor mediated ventilatory response to a step-wise change in $P_{ET}O_2$ had two components: a fast component with a mean time constant of 2 seconds, and a slow component with a mean time constant of 72.6 seconds. Because the studies were in anaesthetised cats, Berkenbosch and his colleagues[1] were able to isolate the peripheral chemoreceptor response by using artificial brain stem perfusion. In humans, however, indirect methods have to be used in an attempt to quantify the peripheral chemoreceptor mediated hypoxic ventilatory response.

Dejours' test[2] has been used as an index of pure peripheral chemoreceptor reflex as it was thought that the stimulus was too short to evoke any central hypoxic effects. We had used a modified Dejour's test (transient hypoxia produced by three breaths of 100% N_2) to assess the peripheral component of the hypoxic ventilatory response in normal subjects. However, studies with the specific chemoreceptor stimulant almitrine[3] showed that almitrine potentiated the ventilatory response to progressive isocapnic hypoxia but did not consistently increase the ventilatory response to transient hypoxia as expected.[4] In addition, we had found that the ventilatory response to similar degrees of hypoxia produced by either transient hypoxia or a rapid-onset step of hypoxia lasting three minutes could not be described by a single linear system.[5] It seems likely that the three minute hypoxic stimulus is also largely mediated by the peripheral chemoreceptors since the secondary decline in ventilation does not generally start until after 5-10 minutes exposure to hypoxia.[6]

Our aim was to develop the simplest model structure relating minute ventilation to ear oxygen saturation in normal subjects in response to both transient and step hypoxic stimuli in order to obtain a better quantitative description of the initial ventilatory response to hypoxia in conscious humans. The assumptions were that oxygen saturation was a measure of the hypoxic stimulus and minute ventilation (V_E) was a measure of the response. The model structure also had to be compatible with an approximately proportional relationship between arterial Hb-oxygen saturation (S_pO_2) and V_E during steady state isocapnic hypoxia.

Development of the model

Experimental data was obtained in 11 normal subjects. All measurements were made during moderate exercise as the raised tidal volume allowed an adequate transient hypoxic stimulus (reduction in ear oxygen saturation to between 80-90%) to be produced with one to three breaths of N_2. The stimulus could therefore be given without the subject's knowledge. Tidal volume (V_T) and respiratory frequency (fR) were recorded and used to calculate

127

instantaneous minute ventilation ($V_E$inst = V_T x fR, l.min^{-1}, BTPS) for each breath. Inspired and end-tidal PO_2 and PCO_2 were also recorded continuously (VG Spectralab-M mass spectrometer). Ear S_PO_2 was measured with a Hewlett-Packard 47201A oximeter adjusted to a time constant of approximately 1.6 seconds.[7] In each subject, the ventilatory response was recorded to a) 6 transient stimuli consisting of one to three breaths of N_2 to reduce S_PO_2 to between 80-85%, b) two step hypoxic stimuli where S_PO_2 was maintained at 90% for three minutes, and c) two step hypoxic stimuli where S_PO_2 was maintained between 80-85% for three minutes. The step hypoxic stimuli were induced with one to three breaths of N_2 to produce a rapid onset. Isocapnia was achieved during the onset and duration of the step stimuli but not during the return to air. The return of ventilation to baseline on the removal of a step hypoxic stimulus was therefore excluded from the model fitting process.

For all models, the input (S) was the depression in saturation from the normoxic level. The output of the model (V) was calculated and compared to the experimentally recorded rise in $V_E$inst. The complexity of the model was increased progessively until a structure was found which adequately fitted all experimental data.

Details of the computer programs, method for assessing relative goodness of fit between the model V and the experimental data, and the method for assessing the precision of the parameter estimation with the final model are given elsewhere.[8]

A single linear differential equation
The simplest model used was a single linear differential equation:

$$ S \quad \rightarrow \boxed{V + \text{tau} \cdot dV/dt = GS} \rightarrow V $$

Tau was the time constant, and G was the gain of the system. Using this model, parameters that gave a good fit between V and $V_E$inst in response to transient hypoxia underestimated the increase in response to step change hypoxia, whereas those giving a good fit for step change hypoxia overestimated the response to transient hypoxia. Thus the two types of hypoxia could not be described adequately by a single linear system confirming our previous observations.[5]

A non-linear differential equation
Since a single linear equation proved inadequate, the next level was to investigate the effect of adding non-linear terms into the single linear differential equation This was done in two ways.
a. Effect of a threshold: The gain was allowed to change at a threshold of S, dS/dt, V, or dV/dt.
b. The gain of the equation was allowed to "saturate" in a manner analogous to the Michaelis-Menton equation:

$$S \rightarrow \boxed{V + tau \cdot dV/dt = GS/(1 + sigma \cdot S)} \rightarrow V$$

where sigma was the coefficient of saturation.

Neither form produced a significantly better fit to the experimental data than the single differential equation.

Two linear differential equations

Various forms of interaction of two linear differential equations were then investigated:

a. an arrangement in series with the output of one equation being the input of the other, and with the output of the second equation forming the overall output:

Equation 1   Equation 2

$$S \rightarrow \boxed{y_1 + tau_1 \cdot dV_1/dt = G_1 \cdot S} \rightarrow \boxed{y_2 + tau_2 \cdot dV/dt = G_2 \cdot S} \rightarrow V$$

b. an arrangement in parallel with both differential equations receiving the same input and with the output of both being summed to give the overall output:

Equation 1

$$y_1 + tau_1 \cdot dy/dt = G_1 \cdot S$$

$$S \qquad\qquad\qquad\qquad\qquad\qquad\qquad\qquad\qquad \rightarrow V$$

Equation 2

$$y_2 + tau_2 \cdot dy/dt = G_2 \cdot S$$

The best fit was consistently obtained using the two equations in parallel with both output summed and with compartment 1 having a fast time constant (< 3sec) and compartment 2 having a slow time constant. However, the slow time constant in equation 2 resulted in a slow return in V to baseline following the transient hypoxic stimulus. The output y_2 was therefore set to zero when $S < 2\%$ to eliminate this effect. Even after elimination of the slow recovery, this model did not adequately describe the data in all subjects. A further level of complexity was therefore required.

Two linear differential equations with non-linear terms

Simple non-linear terms were added to both the two differential equations in parallel. These included (a) the "saturation" term described above, (b) allowing the gain of one equation to depend on the output of the other to simulate inhibition or potentiation, and (c) introducing time delays in different parts of the equations. The simplest model that described the experimental data in all subjects was found to be two linear differential equations in parallel with two additional parameters.

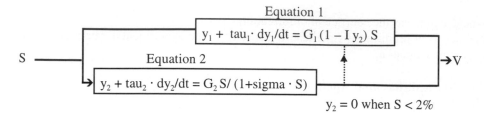

Equation 1

$$y_1 + tau_1 \cdot dy_1/dt = G_1 (1 - I \, y_2) \, S$$

S

Equation 2

$$y_2 + tau_2 \cdot dy_2/dt = G_2 \, S/ (1+sigma \cdot S)$$

→V

$y_2 = 0$ when $S < 2\%$

The equation with the slow time constant (equation 2) contained a "saturation" term as described above. In addition, the output of the equation with the fast time constant (equation 1) was "inhibited" (positive parameter I) or "potentiated" (negative parameter I) by the output of equation 2. The mean values for the parameters which gave the best fit in the 10 normal subjects are given in the table. The fitted values of tau_1 were all < 3 sec. which was less than a breath and therefore could not be measured accurately with the system used.

subject no.	G_1 (l·min^{-1}·%$^{-1}$)	I (l·min^{-1})	tau_2 (s)	G_2 (l·min^{-1}·%$^{-1}$)	sigma (%)
1	3.06	-0.002	59	16.96	1.07
2	0.30	#	29	5.46	#
3	0.19	-2.179	43	34.78	#
4	0.16	#	79	9.74	#
5	0.84	#	66	43.23	4.98
6	4.74	-0.006	9	19.29	#
7	1.60	11.52	196	0.12	#
8	0.20	#	17	3.75	#
9	0.62	-5.071	1318	0.11	#
10	1.29	#	30	95.09	4.67

# indicates parameter not needed for best fit between V and V_E inst

Comment
The model depended on two main assumptions. Firstly, S_PO_2 was taken as a measure of the stimulus. The PO_2 within the glomus cells is considered to be the stimulus to the peripheral chemoreceptors.[9] However, during the rapid onset of the hypoxic stimuli, end-tidal PO_2 will

not accurately reflect arterial P_{O_2}. Subsequent studies which we have done suggest that the models fit less well when a saturation derived from end-tidal P_{O_2} is used as input. Secondly, it was assume that constancy of the end-tidal P_{CO_2} mirrored a constancy in arterial P_{CO_2}, which may not have been true especially during the transient stimuli.

Parameters for individual subjects had wide standard errors.[8] The model structure would therefore need refinement in order to distinguish between subjects. However, it is the model structure which is of interest. We emphasize that the model was developed empirically on a purely mathematical basis. Any physiological interpretation must therefore be treated with considerable caution. Nevertheless, it is interesting that the simplest model that gave the best fit in all 10 normal subjects consisted of two differential equations with the output summed to give the overall ventilatory response. This structure is similar to that described by Berkenbosch and colleagues[1] for their model of the ventilatory response of the peripheral chemoreceptor reflex loop to step changes in P_{O_2}. The short duration of stimuli which we used (transient and three minute step changes) should avoid any central effect of hypoxia and the ventilatory response should therefore reflect the peripheral chemoreceptor reflex. If this is the case, then our model suggests that in conscious humans, as in anaesthetised cats, the peripheral chemoreceptor response contains a fast and a slow component.

References
1. Berkenbosch A, DeGoede J, Ward DS, Olievier CN, VanHartevelt J. Dynamic response of the peripheral chemoreflex loop to changes in end-tidal O_2. *J Appl Physiol* 71: 1123-28, 1991.
2. Dejours P. La regulation de la ventilation au cours de l'exercise musculaire chez l'homme. *J Physiol (Paris)* 51: 163-261, 1953.
3. Laubie N, Schmitt H. Long-lasting hyperventilation induced by almitrine: evidence for a specific effect on carotid and thoracic chemoreceptors. *Eur J Pharm* 61: 125-36, 1980.
4 Airlie MMA, Flenley DC, Warren PM. Effect of almitrine on hypoxic ventilatory drive measured by transient and progressive isocapnic hypoxia in normal men. *Clin Sci* 77: 431-37, 1989.
5. Warren PM, Airlie MAA, De Cort SC, Kirby TP, Wraith PK, Flenley DC. The ventilatory response to hypoxia is a function of the rate of change of the stimulus. *Am Rev Respir Dis* 135 (suppl): A369, 1987.
6. Easton PA, Slykerman LJ, Anthonisen NR. Ventilatory response to sustained hypoxia in normal adults. *J Appl Physiol* 61: 906-11, 1986.
7. Douglas NJ, Brash HM, Wraith PK, Calverley PMA, Leggett RJ, McElderry L, Flenley DC. Accuracy, sensitivity to carbon monoxide, and speed of response of the Hewlett-Packard 47201A ear oximeter. *Am Rev Respir Dis* 119: 311-3, 1979
8. Kirby TP, Wraith PK, De Cort SC, Airlie MAA, Hill JE, Carson ER, Flenley DC, Warren PM. Modelling the dynamic ventilatory response to hypoxia in normal subjects. *J Theoret Biol* 166: 135-47, 1994.
9. Ezyguirre C, Zapata P. Perspectives in carotid body research. *J Appl Physiol* 57: 931-57, 1984.

Some theoretical consequences of a linear ventilatory response to both hypoxia and hypercapnia

Peter A. Robbins

Introduction

The ventilatory response to hypercapnia is generally considered linear for values of end-tidal PCO_2 greater than normal.[1] Similarly, there is a notion that there exists some function of PO_2, termed hypoxia, to which ventilation responds linearly. Several forms have been suggested for this function, and these include a hyperbolic form, an exponential form, and a form based on the saturation of haemoglobin that would arise from the level of PO_2.[2] The slope of the relation between ventilation and hypercapnia is dependent on the level of hypoxia, and similarly the slope of the relation between ventilation and hypoxia is dependent on the level of hypercapnia.

The ventilatory response to hypercapnia at different constant levels of hypoxia is generally drawn as a set of lines with a common point of origin, often referred to as the "Oxford fan". However, it is not immediately obvious that there necessarily should be a common point of intersection for all the lines. Indeed, it is certainly possible to draw a set of straight lines for the ventilatory response to hypercapnia where there is no common point of intersection. In this paper, it is shown that, if the ventilatory response to hypercapnia at constant hypoxia is linear, and if the response to hypoxia at constant hypercapnia is linear, then there must be a common point of intersection for the hypercapnic response lines and also a common point of intersection for the hypoxic response lines. There are a number of corollaries to this. First, if experimentally it is shown that there is no common point of intersection for, say, the hypercapnic response lines, then there does not exist any function of PO_2 for which the ventilatory response will be linear for all levels of PCO_2. Secondly, apart from any parameters used in defining hypoxia and hypercapnia, the ventilatory response can be described completely in its most general form using four parameters. Finally, it is also shown that if, say, all the hypercapnic response lines do intersect at a common point, then there is some function of PO_2, hypoxia, to which ventilation is linearly related at constant hypercapnia and that these lines intersect at a common point.

This paper has been presented in terms of ventilatory responses to hypercapnia and hypoxia. However, the results are equally valid for studies of the response of the carotid body to hypercapnia and hypoxia (e.g. Lahiri and DeLaney)[3].

Theorem

Let x be the hypercapnic stimulus function, where $x: PCO_2 \mapsto x(PCO_2)$, and y be the hypoxic stimulus function, where $y: PO_2 \mapsto y(PO_2)$. Let v be the steady-state ventilatory control function, where $v: (x(PCO_2), y(PO_2)) \mapsto v(x(PCO_2), y(PO_2))$. If $\partial v / \partial x = f(y)$, and

$\partial v / \partial y = g(x)$, then $v(x,y) = a (x + b) (y + c) + d$, where, a, b, c and d are constants.

Proof

$$\partial v / \partial x = f(y) \Rightarrow v = f(y) \cdot x + m(y) \Rightarrow \partial v / \partial y = f'(y) \cdot x + m'(y)$$

where m is an arbitrary function of y. Also,

$$\partial v / \partial y = g(x) \Rightarrow v = g(x) \cdot y + n(x) \Rightarrow \partial v / \partial x = g'(x) \cdot y + n'(x)$$

where n is an arbitrary function of x. Hence,

$$\partial v / \partial x = f(y) = g'(x) \cdot y + n'(x) \Rightarrow g'(x) = k_1 \text{ and } n'(x) = k_2$$

where k_1 and k_2 are constants. Also,

$$\partial v / \partial y = g(x) = f'(y) \cdot x + m'(y) \Rightarrow f'(y) = k_3 \text{ and } \Rightarrow m'(y) = k_4$$

where k_3 and k_4 are constants. Substitution yields $f(y) = k_1 y + k_2$ and $g(x) = k_3 x + k_4$, and integrating yields $n(x) = k_3 x + k_4$, and $m(y) = k_4 y + k_6$, where k_5 and k_6 are constants. Substituting either the expressions for $g(x)$ and $n(x)$ or the expressions for $f(y)$ and $m(y)$ into one of the expressions obtained for v yields the form of the response. Using $g(x)$ and $n(x)$,

$$v = (k_3 x + k_4) y + k_2 x + k_5$$

$$v = k_3 x y + k_2 x + k_4 y + k_5$$

$$v = k_3 (x + (k_4 / k_3)) (y + (k_2 / k_3)) - k_4 k_2 / k_3 + k_5$$

$$v = a(x + b) (y + c) + d$$

where $a = k_3$, $b = k_4 / k_3$, $c = k_2 / k_3$ and $d = k_5 - k_2 k_4 / k_3$.

Discussion

In the theorem, a hypercapnic stimulus function, x, has been defined. However, the ventilatory response is considered by most to be linear with PCO_2 , consequently the function x can become just the identity function $x : PCO_2 \mapsto PCO_2$. In some ways the hypercapnic stimulus function is thus an unnecessary complication, but it was included in the proof for the sake of completeness and for symmetry with the hypoxic stimulus function.

One of the major physiological points arising from the theorem is that the question of whether the stimulus response lines meet at a single point or not when extrapolated to lower values of PCO_2 is relevant to our understanding of the response at *normal and elevated* PCO_2, and not just to ideas concerning chemoreceptor thresholds (e.g. Cunningham[4]).

Consequently, if we are to find any function of hypoxia to which ventilation responds linearly (the slope dependent only on the PCO_2), then it is necessary for the hypercapnic response lines to meet at a single point.

Another physiological point that arises from the theorem is that, if the ventilation is going to respond linearly to both hypercapnia and hypoxia, then the most general form of the equation is $v = a(x + b)(y + c) + d$. This equation is of the same form as that described in Severinghaus' review,[2] but the additional conclusion that now follows is that there is no more general equation compatible with linear responses to both hypercapnia and hypoxia.

A final point to be drawn is that, if the extrapolations of the hypercapnic response lines do indeed meet at a single point, then there does exist some hypoxic function of PO_2 such that the ventilatory response to hypoxia is always linear at any constant PCO_2. This may be seen from the fact that the most general equation for a set of hypercapnic response lines through a common point (v_1, x_1) is given by

$$v - v_1 = m(PO_2)(x - x_1)$$

where $m(PO_2)$ is the slope of the relation between v and PCO_2, and can depend only on the PO_2. By inspection, however, the equation also represents a linear response to $m(PO_2)$ of slope $(x - x_1)$. Hence $m(PO_2)$ is a suitable hypoxic function (y), and by the theorem (since the responses to both hypercapnia and hypoxia are linear) the v $m(PO_2)$ response lines must also meet at a common point.

References

1. Cunningham DJC, Robbins PA, Wollf CB. Integration of respiratory responses to changes in alveolar partial pressures of CO_2 and O_2 and in arterial *pH*. In: *Handbook of Physiology: The Respiratory System, vol 2*. Edited by Cherniack NS and Widdicombe JG. Bethesda, MD, USA, American Physiological Society, pp 475-528, 1986.
2. Severinghaus JW. Proposed standard determination of ventilatory responses to hypoxia and hypercapnia in man. *Chest* 70 (suppl): 129-131, 1976.
3. Lahiri S, DeLaney RG. Stimulus interaction in the responses of carotid body chemoreceptor single afferent fibres. *Respir Physiol* 24: 267-286, 1975.
4. Cunningham, DJC. Integrative aspects of the regulation of breathing: a personal view. In: *Respiration Physiology, series 1, vol 2, MTP International Review of Science*. Edited by Guyton AC and Widdicombe JG. London, UK, Butterworth, pp 303-370, 1974.

The Read method to assess ventilatory regulation

J.M. Bogaard

Since 1967 the Read method became a popular approach for the estimation of ventilatory CO_2 sensitivity.[1,2] The method is quick and easy. A 4 to 6 liter rebreathing bag is filled with 7% CO_2 in oxygen. If the patient rebreathes for about 4 minutes a marked increase in ventilation occurs which, together with the linear rise in end-tidal PCO_2 ($PetCO_2$), gives the CO_2 sensitivity.

Read and co-workers interpreted the results as follows: due to the initial concentration of CO_2 in the bag a quick equilibrium of CO_2 exchange occurs with the $PetCO_2$ level near mixed venous PCO_2 ($PvCO_2$). Then arterial PCO_2 ($PaCO_2$), $PetCO_2$ and $PvCO_2$ and presumably brain tissue PCO_2 ($PtCO_2$) all start to increase with the same rate of rise. Because the central CO_2 sensitivity is located within cerebral tissue, $PtCO_2$ is assumed to be the stimulus and therefore the $PetCO_2$ vs. ventilation increase is assumed to be a valid CO_2 sensitivity index. Berkenbosch et al.[3] and Dahan et al.[4] convincingly showed, theoretically and experimentally, that the Read method markedly overestimates the steady-state ventilatory CO_2 response. In figure 1 experimentally obtained results are presented in which the steady-state estimate is obtained from a stepwise increase in $PetCO_2$, keeping this value constant for 8 min.[3] The larger rebreathing ventilatory carbon dioxide sensitivity compared to the steady-state ventilatory carbon dioxide sensitivity is explained by the large increase in cerebral blood flow due to the $PaCO_2$ increase. This was already shown in 1948 by Kety and Schmidt.[5] In the steady state this causes a decrease in the $PaCO_2$-$PtCO_2$ gradient in the cerebral tissue causing a decrease in the rise of the real stimulus compared to the measured stimulus ($PetCO_2$).

Dahan et al.[4] theoretically analyzed the mass balance for CO_2 as was already proposed by Read and Leigh[2] and Berkenbosch et al.[3] Changes in $PtCO_2$ were analyzed in relation to changes in $PaCO_2$ defined by an initial $PetCO_2$ step (A) and a linear rate of rise (R). Parameters in the mass balance equation were: brain blood flow density (Q'), brain metabolism (M'), the slopes of the blood and brain CO_2 dissociation curves and the location of the chemoreceptor sites (with $PtCO_2$ as stimulus) between $PaCO_2$ and cerebral venous PCO_2. A and R can be chosen such that the rise in $PtCO_2$ equals that in $PaCO_2$ (or $PetCO_2$). These conditions were called "Read conditions". In figure 2 examples are given for theoretically obtained deviations from the steady-state CO_2 sensitivity (Ss; Sn/Ss) in relation to parameter A, in case of a constant value of R (0.5 kPa/min) and four different combinations of M' and Q'_0 (initial brain blood flow density) values. The figure shows that only specific conditions of A and R yield an Ss estimate with appreciable accuracy. Another approach for the estimation of the "Read conditions" by Smit et al.[6] was based on the dynamic changes of ventilation (V_1) after a step of $PetCO_2$, as obtained by the dynamic

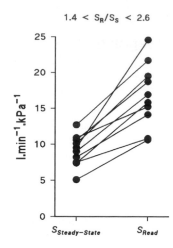

Figure 1. Comparison of the Read and steady-state ventilatory response on the ventilatory CO_2 sensitivty in 10 normal volunteers. S_S is the CO_2 sensitivity obtained with the steady-state method, S_R the CO_2 sensitivity from rebreathing. (adapted from ref. 3).

end-tidal forcing (DEF) technique, described by DeGoede et al .[7] A step change of PetCO$_2$ causes a stimulus of both central and peripheral chemoreceptors, resulting in a contribution of both stimulus sites to ventilatory output. The differential equation, describing the dynamics of the system resulted in two additive single-exponential ventilation increases, the contribution of the peripheral chemoreceptors with a small and that of the central chemoreceptors with a larger time constant.

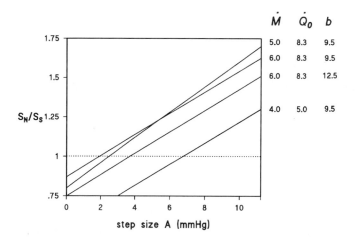

Figure 2. Theoretical prediction of the relation between the ratio of "pseudo-Read" and steady state CO_2 sensitivity (S_N and S_S, respectively) and PetCO$_2$ step (A) in case of a ramp slope of 0.5 kPa·min^{-1}. The relation is shown for four combinations of M' and Q'o. M' brain metabolism (units 10^{-4} ml·ml^{-1}·s^{-1}), Q'$_0$ initial brain blood flow density (units 10^{-3} ml·ml^{-1}·s^{-1}); adapted from ref. 4.

Berkenbosch et al.[4] solved the differential equation for a step-ramp input of $PetCO_2$ and they derived the equation:

$$Sd(t)/Ss = [(A/sTc- 1) / (1 + a)] \ exp -[(t - Tc)/Tc] \qquad (1)$$

with

Sd(t)	=	time dependent deviation from Ss
Ss	=	steady state CO_2 sensitivity
Tc	=	time constant V_I output by central chemoreceptors
Tc	=	time delay chemoreceptor stimulus
Gp	=	gain of peripheral chemoreflex loop
Gc	=	gain of central chemoreflex loop
Gp/Gc	=	a

Smit et al.[6] derived from the literature, among others from Dahan et al.[8] representative values for the indices in humans. These values were Gp/Gc = 0.15, Tc 0.20 min, Tc = 1.65 min. Because in eqn. 1 it is assumed that after 20 s the peripheral exponential term becomes negligible the peripheral chemoreceptor influence is not taken into account. The equation was solved for two different procedures, firstly for a step of about 5% CO_2 and a ramp slope of 0.4 kPa·min^{-1} (step-ramp, SR procedure) and secondly for a procedure with a ramp slope of 0.2 kPa·min^{-1} without an initial step (R procedure).

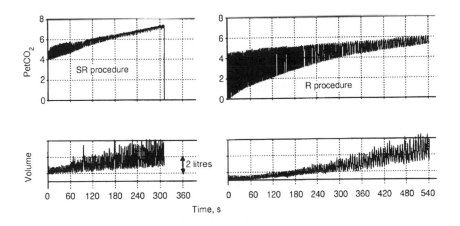

Figure 3. Representative time course of $PetCO_2$ and minute volume, as recorded by spirometry, during SR and R procedure (with permission from ref. 6).

For the SR procedure this was accomplished in practice by rebreathing in a spirometer system with 10 l of 5% CO_2 in 50% O_2 in which the sodalime absorber was removed. In the R procedure partial CO_2 absorption was used to obtain the desired ramp slope. In figure 3 two representative time courses of $PetCO_2$ and V_I for the SR and R approach are given, respectively. Although a closed loop situation was present the ramp slopes appeared to be linear in good approximation.

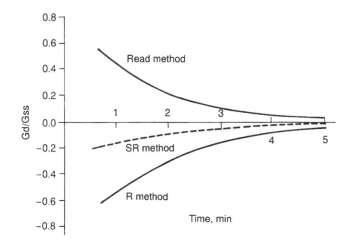

Figure 4. Predicted ratio for the hyperoxic condition between the SR, R and classical Read CO_2 sensitivity estimate and the steady-state value. See further the text (with permission from ref. 6).

Furthermore, figure 4 shows the theoretical prediction, based on equation 1, of the time dependent deviation from Ss. Using the original Read values the prediction indeed gave an overestimation of about 20-30% over the first 4 minutes. The SR approach gave a slight underestimation and the prediction leads to the use of the data from 0.5 to 8 min from the start of the rebreathing procedure. The R method showed no appreciable deviation, starting from the fifth minute which leads to the use of the data of the four last minutes of the 8 minutes lasting rebreathing procedure. In 12 volunteers indeed a similar ventilatory response on CO_2 was found for the last four minutes of the R and for the whole SR procedure, omitting the first 0.5 min (12.5 ± 7.0 and 13.0 ± 4.6 l.min^{-1}.kPa^{-1} respectively).

It is interesting to realize that Hirschman et al.[8] proposed a similar R procedure in which they, for experimental reasons, also used the data from the last part of the procedure.

From the work of Berkenbosch et al.[3], Dahan et al.[4] and Smit et al.[6] it can be concluded that the classical Read-method has to be replaced by a Read like approach in which step and ramp slope are carefully chosen.

References
1. Read DJC. A clinical method for assessing the ventilatory response to carbon dioxide. *Australas Ann Med* 16: 20 - 32, 1967.
2. Read DJC, Leigh J. Blood-brain tissue PCO_2 relationships and ventilation during rebreathing. *J Appl Physiol* 23: 53 - 70, 1967.
3. Berkenbosch A, Bovill JG, Dahan A, Goede J de, Olivier ICW. The ventilatory CO_2 sensitivities from Read's rebreathing method and the steady state method are not equal in man. *J Physiol* 411: 367 - 377, 1989.
4. Dahan A, Berkenbosch A, Goede J de, Olivier CN, Bovill JG. On a pseudo-rebreathing technique to assess the ventilatory sensitivity to carbon dioxide in man. *J Physiol* 423: 615 - 629, 1990.
5. Kety SS, Schmidt CF. The effects of altered arterial tension of carbon dioxide and oxygen on cerebral blood flow and cerebral oxygen consumption of normal man. *J Clin Invest* 27: 484 - 492, 1948.
6. Smit JM, Bogaard JM, Goorden G, Verbraak AFM, Dalinghaus P. A Quasi Steady State Ramp Method for the Estimation of the ventilatory Response to CO_2. *Respiration* 59: 9 - 15, 1992.
7. Goede J de, Berkenbosch A, Ward DS, Belville JW, Olivier CN. Comparison of the chemoreflex gains with two different methods in cats. *J Appl Physiol* 59: 170 - 179, 1985.
8. Dahan A, Goede J de, Berkenbosch A, Olivier CN. The influence of oxygen on the ventilatory response to carbon dioxide in man. *J Physiol* 428: 485 - 499, 1990.
9. Hirschman CA, McCullough RE, Weil JV. Normal values for hypoxic and hypercapnic ventilatory drives in man. *J Appl Physiol* 38: 1095 - 1098, 1975.

Index terms arranged per chapter

p 45 End-tidal inspiratory activity ....

Airway pressure
Asthma
Clinical study
End-tidal inspiratory activity
Histamine
Hyperinflation
Lung, receptors

p 51 Sleep disordered breathing ....

Clinical study
COPD
Control of breathing
Hypoxia
Lung, disease
Sleep
Sleep related disorders

p 59 Sleep apnea syndrome ....

Autonomic nervous system
Control of breathing
Clinical study
Respiratory oscillations
Sleep
Sleep apnea
Sleep related disorders

p 65 Children who forget ....

Autonomic nervous system
Congenital hypoventilation syndrome
Newborn
Control of breathing
Sleep
Sleep related disorders
Wakefulness

146

p 93 Opioid-induced analgesia and

Analgesia
Analgesia, spinal, supraspinal
Animal study
Control of breathing
Morphine
Nociception
Opioid, receptors
Opioid, receptors, mu, kappa, delta
Sex differences
Sex hormones

p 101 Separate effects of respiratory stimuli ....

Control of breathing
Diaphragm
Fentanyl
Human study
Hypercapnia
Hypoxia
Lung
Opioids
Respiratory muscles

p 109 Influences of low dose ....

Anesthesia
Anesthetics, volatile
Carotid body
Chemoreceptors
Control of breathing
Hypercapnia
Hypoxia
Knill, Richard
Methodology
Ventilatory response to hypercapnia
Ventilatory response to hypoxia

148

p 115 Cardiovascular and pulmonary ......

Anesthesia
Anesthetics
Animal study
Cardiac output
Cardiovadcular responses
Lung
Lung uptake
Modelling
Pharmacokinetics

p 121 Pharmacokinetic-Pharmacodynamic modeling ......

Anesthesia
Anesthetics, volatile
Animal study
Control of breathing
Modelling
PK-PD Modelling
Sevoflurane

p 127 An empirical model .....

Human study
Hypoxia
Modelling
Ventilatory response to hypoxia

p 133 Some theoretical consequences .....

Control of breathing
Hypoxia
Hypercapnia
Modelling
Oxford-fan

p 137 The Read method to .....

Human study
Control of breathing
Methodology
Modelling
Rebreathing
Ventilatory response to carbon dioxide